LONDON PRIDE

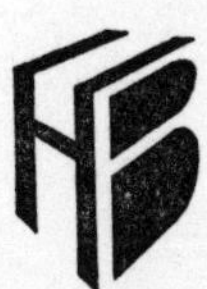

By the same author

Stephen Hales: an Eighteenth Century Biography
Edith Cavell, Pioneer and Patriot
Attack the Colour:
The Royal Dragoons in the Peninsula and at Waterloo
Man, Medicine and Morality
Medicine in its Human Setting
Patients as People
How to Learn Medicine
Lectures on Medicine to Nurses

LONDON PRIDE

The story of a voluntary hospital

A. E. CLARK-KENNEDY

HUTCHINSON BENHAM
LONDON

Hutchinson Benham Limited
3 Fitzroy Square, London W 1P 6JD

An imprint of the Hutchinson Group

London Melbourne Sydney Auckland
Wellington Johannesburg and agencies
throughout the world

First published 1979
© The London Hospital Special Trustees 1979

Set in Monotype Bembo

Printed in Great Britain by The Anchor Press Ltd
and bound by Wm Brendon & Son Ltd
both of Tiptree, Essex

British Library Cataloguing in Publication Data
Clark-Kennedy, Archibald Edmund
   London Pride
   1. London Hospital and Medical College – History
   I. Title
   362.1'1'094215   RA988.L8L/

ISBN 0 09 136541 4

*To the memory of Sydney Holland,
second Viscount Knutsford*

Contents

Preface

Thirty years have now passed since the voluntary hospitals were taken over by the state, and it seems almost forgotten that from the Reformation up to 1870 – when the Poor Law Board admitted 'that the sick were not a proper object for the deterrent system' – the care of the poor *in hospital* depended on charity. Up to the First World War they remained largely dependent on it; dependent on it up to a point until the National Health Act came into force in 1948 and senior medical staff started to be paid.

The story of many of them has been told for the benefit of those who have served them, and, early in the sixties, I wrote a history of my own hospital, 'the London', from its foundation in 1740 up to its acquisition by the state in 1948. In this I endeavoured to tell its story, not in isolation, but in relation to historical events, social change and the many problems it had to face created by the growth of science and technology.*

My two volumes are now out of print, and in this one-volume edition I have cut out much only of interest to 'old Londoners' and concentrated on the problems which were common to all the hospitals and on those particular episodes in our history of interest to the general reader. On 'the text' of 'the London' I have in fact endeavoured to tell the story of the voluntary system as a whole, of its achievement as an episode in history and of its triumph as charitable endeavour.

* *The London: a Study in the Voluntary Hospital System*, 2 vol., Pitman Medical Publishing Company, London, 1961 and 1963.

As my two original volumes are accessible in libraries, I thought it unnecessary to reprint references to the sources on which my book is based. All quotations, unless otherwise stated, are from the minutes of the board of governors and are transcribed as written, regardless of grammar, spelling, punctuation and use of capital letters.

To the inspiration of John Ellis MBE, MD, FRCP, at one time my student and then my house physician, later my sub-dean, and now senior physician to the hospital and my second successor as dean of the medical college, I am indebted for the title which I have ventured to adopt for this book.

A. E. CLARK-KENNEDY

December 1978

Prologue

The medieval church, out of the spirit of Christian charity, had shouldered the burden of the poor for centuries, and when Henry VIII suppressed the religious houses their plight must have been heartrending. Suddenly there was nowhere for the sick to look for help or for the aged to seek asylum. So the Lord Mayor and citizens of London had implored the King to re-found the priory of St Bartholomew in Smithfield and that of St Thomas across London Bridge in Southwark 'for the ayde and comfort of the poore sikke, blynde, aged and impotent persones, beyng not able to helpe theymselffs, nor hauyning any place certeyn whereyn they may be lodged, cherysshed and refresshed tyll they be cured and holpen of theyre dyseases and syckesse'. If only the King would grant them back these hospitals, they would be reformed, they promised – there were many stories about them – and their usefulness increased.

This appeal fell on a stony heart. Not for six years did the King respond, and then half-heartedly. St Bartholomew's was now reconstituted by royal favour under a master and four chaplains with lay sisters to care for the sick. But provision on this scale for the whole of London was quite inadequate and, in the last year of his life, Henry was forced into more generous action. He agreed to endow St Bartholomew's to the tune of £330 per annum, and the citizens of London, thinking this 'rather too little than enough', raised nearly £1000 to enable the hospital to provide a hundred beds. St Bartholomew's was in fact re-founded on a secular basis, not so much out of the spoliation of the monasteries as out of the pockets of the more wealthy citizens of London, and the charter, granted by the King, put it virtually under the jurisdiction of the City. 'In consequence,' writes D'Arcy Power, 'the Charity, which had been free to all at its foundation, became obstructed by a system of Governors' letters and even after admission (by governor's letter) fees of various kinds were demanded of patients.' Before he died the King also gave St Mary's of Bethlehem (where Liverpool Street Station now stands) to the City as 'a hospital for distracted people'. This was hedged about with similar restrictions.

In the next reign the City, encouraged by the success of their St Bartholomew's venture, purchased the Manor of Southwark and reopened St Thomas's Hospital. Edward VI himself founded Bridewell as a 'House of Correction and Workhouse for the poor, for the strumpet, for the idle person, for the rioter that consumeth all and for the vagabond that will abide no place'. Then this thin stream of refoundation dried up. The opportunity of using money derived from the spoliation of the monasteries for starting municipal hospitals had been missed. The Elizabethan Poor Law was to provide domiciliary medicine, and some workhouses sick wards for their own paupers, but throughout the rest of the sixteenth and the whole of the seventeenth century London continued without other hospitals.

Meanwhile, its population went on increasing, partly due to the incursion of refugees from the Continent, partly due to the importation of cheap labour from Ireland, and partly due to a rise in the birth-rate, with the result that, by the beginning of the eighteenth century, the condition of the sick poor was deplorable. Before long the social conscience had been stirred. In 1713 Addison of the *Guardian* pointed to the need for a hospital for children abandoned by their mothers, an article which inspired Captain Coram to raise money for the Foundling Hospital in Guilford Street. In 1720 four gentlemen of evangelical persuasion collected subscriptions and opened the Westminster Infirmary in Petty France, a number of fashionable physicians and surgeons offering their services in an honorary capacity. A year later

Mr Guy, a governor of St Thomas's Hospital who had made a fortune out of South Sea stock and printing Bibles, petitioned his board of governors for ground on which to build a hospital for the incurable. Four years later St Bartholemew's was rebuilt by public subscription. In 1733 St George's Hospital opened in Lanesborough House just outside the Toll Gate, now Hyde Park Corner.

There were now five hospitals in London maintained and supported by voluntary contribution: one in the City, two, in effect, in Southwark, one in the royal borough of Westminster, and a fifth out in the still open country to the west. As yet no hospital had been started to serve the rapidly developing East End, its population swollen by Huguenots in Spitalfields, immigrant Jews in Bethnal Green, and the increasing demand for manpower in London's rapidly expanding docks. For a foundation of this kind the stage was set. This hospital, when it came, was destined, from very small and very humble beginnings, to become the largest and one of the leading hospitals in London.

I

Birth and Infancy

The winter of 1739–40 had been hard, one of the most severe in the whole eighteenth century. The wheat sown in the autumn had been destroyed by frost; the streets of London were blocked by snow; navigation on the river was rendered impossible by ice. There had been more distress among the poor than ever, but many were at last becoming conscious of the needs of the sick, among them a group of professional and business friends: Fotherley Baker, a lawyer and a member of the Haberdashers' Company; Mr Josiah Cole, an apothecary; Shute Adams, the druggist in Fleet Street; Mr John Harrison, a practising surgeon who had been apprenticed to James Ferne of St Thomas's Hospital at fourteen and was still only twenty-three; Mr Sclater, Mr John Snee and Mr G. Potter. There is no evidence that they belonged to any particular religious denomination, as in the case of the founders of the Westminster and St George's before them, but they, too, had been thinking in terms of starting a new hospital. On 23 September 1740 they foregathered in the Feathers Tavern in Cheapside, the first meeting of the subscribers to 'an intended new Infirmary'.

Sclater was chosen as chairman, Fotherley Baker elected treasurer. Weekly meetings were to be held and minutes kept. Then, we are told, 'Mr Harrison delivered in the Lease of the House for the Infirmary, whereupon it was proposed that the several Subscriptions made to compleat the Sum of 100 Guineas be produced next Tuesday.' This settled, 'a Motion was made

Whether with the Sum already Subscribed it would be proper to begin the said Charity? And unanimously agreed it was.' St Bartholomew's had been re-founded by the King and St Thomas's by the City, the Westminster and St George's started by evangelicals, and Guy's endowed by one rich man. 'The London' owes its origin to seven ordinary men meeting in a public house, the leading spirit among them John Harrison, a member of the Barber Surgeons' Company.

The house which he had secured at £16 per annum stood in Featherstone Street, just outside Moor Gate, a turning out of Royal Row, now City Road. It was to open in little more than a month, so a number of practical matters had to be settled. 'The first Business proceeded to', run the minutes of their next meeting, 'was the providing of a Man and Woman proper to look after the House and attend the Surgeon and Physician, and when Mr Harrison acquainted the Chairman he had spoke to two Persons whom he thought Proper for the Business who were attending below who, being ordered to be called in, They agreed to do all the Business of the said Infirmary for the sum of twenty pounds p.Ann.' Then it was resolved that 'Mr John Harrison and Mr G. Potter do provide furniture for the Physician's, Surgeon's, Apothecary's, Manager's and Patients' Rooms not exceeding the sum of fifteen pounds, and that the Treasurer do pay the Bills for the Same.'

A week later at the Baptist's Head Tavern in Aldermanbury the staff were elected: Dr Andrée, M.D. of Rheims, a Huguenot refugee, to be the physician, Harrison and Cole, as was to be expected, surgeon and apothecary respectively. The subscribers also decided to keep a book in which to record in several columns 'the Names of the Patients, their Business and Place of Abode, Disorder, the Issue of the Case, and the Name of the Subscriber who sent them'. Then they applied themselves to roping in new subscribers and agreed to send out two thousand letters with this intent. For the money side of things was not going well. A margin note in red in the minutes of this meeting, and in the same hand as that which wrote them, reads: '1s. in Bank.'

Nevertheless, the London Hospital, or Infirmary as it was first called, did open its doors, as planned, on 3 November 1740 and, when the subscribers met again, this time at the Black Swan in Bartholomew Lane, John Harrison reported that the Duke of Richmond had sent a subscription and that there was hope of obtaining others from 'Persons of Quality and Distinction'. (The patronage of the nobility was essential to the success of any middle-class venture in those days.) The subscribers then approved draft rules for patients attending the infirmary and authorized the treatment of maternity cases as out-patients. 'Mr Cole, the Apothecary to this Infirmary, also following the Practice of Midwifery, having proposed to attend every Wednesday from 3 to 5 for the Relief of Women with Child and the Distempers incident thereto, Agreed that he do attend accordingly, and give them the necessary Advice and Relief.'

Before long the subscribers had become too large a body to run the daily affairs of the charity, so a committee was appointed 'to attend every Thursday at the Infirmary to inspect and Examine into its Management'. The subscribers continued to meet as a body at intervals at the Black Swan or the Angel and Crown in Aldgate until 'it was considered Improper to hold meetings at Taverns', and Mr Fotherley Baker offered the use of the Haberdashers' Hall for this purpose. Cases of venereal disease, it was agreed, should be treated, but 'so as not to admit them into the House'. The remuneration of the apothecary was fixed. The physician and surgeon gave their services free. Most important of all, the subscribers formally reserved to themselves the sole right of recommending patients for treatment but agreed 'that upon all Extraordinary Accidents and Disorders the Treasurer or the Chairman of the Committee may be at Liberty to direct such Patients to be received into the House whose Cases require it Immediately'.

Within six months the house was proving too small for the purpose for which it was intended, and the treasurer secured the lease of a larger one in Prescott Street in Goodmans Fields just outside the City. This district was the site of many cheap places of low entertainment, forced out by the authorities: the notorious New Wells Theatre, Odell's Playhouse in Great Alie Street and the Turk's Head Bagnio in Ayliff Street. 'To those plays and interludes,' wrote the Justices of the Peace in 1751, 'great numbers of mean, idle and disorderly people do resort, and from thence go to the bawdy houses and the other houses of ill fame near the Wells and Playhouse which are chiefly supported by the concourse of such idle and unwary people as the said plays and interludes draw together greatly to the corruption of the morals of His Majesty's Subjects and the Breach of the Peace.'

The actual move to Prescott Street took place in May. Again, there were many urgent matters to be settled. The house in Moorfields, which had only been occupied for a few months, was put up to let. An apothecary's shop was bought 'from Mr Harris of Ayliff Street for £14 10s. 0d. according to the Inventory delivered'; Mr Cole was ordered to fit it up, with one of his assistants to reside in the house. Twenty-four new beds were ordered and 'some Chairs of Virginia Walnut Tree with matted Seats, not exceeding 6 gns. per Chair for the Doctor's room and two not exceeding 4/6 for the Dispensary'. A 'beautiful and necessary Gown' was presented by Mr Myre, and a staff, in the same exalted category, by Mr Fordham, for the porter. The chairman was instructed 'to see on what Terms the Infirmary could be served by the Brewer, Baker, Butcher, Butterman, Cheesemonger and Milkman'.

Soon after this the subscribers succeeded in getting their charity constituted. Those of five guineas a year became governors; of thirty guineas, in a lump sum, life governors. Any physician or surgeon elected to the staff became a governor. A court of governors was to meet quarterly, peers and ladies to be entitled to send other governors as proxies to vote for them. The court was to elect a house committee to run the day-to-day affairs of the infirmary and report at each meeting.

This committee met at 11 a.m. on Thursdays, any member arriving late being required to put a shilling in the poor box. First the patients '*presented* cured by the Physician' followed by those '*presented* cured by the Surgeon' were called in and required 'to render thanks to their Benefactors' and exhorted to go to their parish churches to return thanks to God 'for the cures they had received at the hands of the Charity'. Any patient who refused to return thanks was never to be treated again (a black list was kept). Those who conformed were given a certificate entitling them to further relief should they ever need it. Then the committee adjourned to the Angel and Crown 'for the better transacting of the Business of the Charity'.

The right to recommend patients for treatment encouraged many local tradesmen and others to subscribe and become governors – it was not altruism alone that did it – and it soon became necessary to ration them: each governor was allowed only one in the house at any time. Exceptions were made when social influence and medical interest coincided. 'George King, recommended by the Rt Hon. the Earl of Buckingham, by Order of the Committee admitted an in-patient, although his Lordship has another patient in the Hospital, his case being very Extraordinary.'

'Accidental' and 'extraordinary' cases (we would call them accidents and acute cases) were admitted at any hour of the day or night. All others were required to present themselves on a committee day armed with a letter of recommendation from a governor. Then the committee, having inquired into their means, took responsibility for accepting or rejecting them. This system involved the committee in a lot of work. Many patients were sent up unnecessarily and before long they had to write round to all the governors 'praying them only to send up such Cases as were *really* Necessitous'. Sometimes, too, a governor would send a seriously ill patient up from the country without finding out in advance if there was a bed for him. Then he might have to be sent home at the expense of the charity.

The committee was also soon faced with the problem of compromising between the rights of the increasing numbers of governors and the continuing needs of the sick poor on their doorstep, most of whom had no means of getting a letter of recommendation from a governor. So a system was introduced by which, on payment of a penny, anyone could petition to be treated and appear before the committee. This penny was often returned. 'During the last Quarter,' the committee reported, 'great numbers of real poor necessitous Objects labouring under the most malignant and deplorable Diseases destitute of friends and means to obtain a Cure otherwise than by such charitable institution as the Infirmary have been restored to Health and Strength and enabled to work and maintain themselves and their poor Families, many of which poor Objects have gratefully and joyously acknowledged the great Benefits they have received from the Charity and prayed to God for their kind Benefactors.'*

Dr Andrée and Mr Harrison started work at 11 a.m., by which time all patients recommended for treatment were required to be present, bringing with them 'Fillets for bleeding and Phyalls or Gallipots to receive their medicines'. Then they went round the wards accompanied by the apothecary and their pupils. For 'the London' started taking pupils early in its existence, the first entering within six months of its foundation. 'Mr Harrison, desiring to enter Mr Godfrey Webb as a pupil for the space of one Year, it was ordered that he be so entered on the Books and that, if he be constantly attendant on the practice of the Infirmary, he shall have a Certificate signifying his Attendance from the Weekly Committee of the Infirmary.' Before starting he was summoned before the committee and enjoined 'to be Constant in his attendance, Tender and Careful to his Patients'. The first pupil in 'physick', Mr Cullen, started at the request of Dr Andrée in 1747.

The committee had some difficulty in finding a nobleman to become president of the infirmary but the Duke of Richmond eventually consented and took the chair at the first meeting of the court of governors under the new constitution. This was held in the hall of the Haberdashers' Company on 12 May 1742, when Mr Fotherley Baker, as vice-president, 'informed the Gentlemen of the several Transactions and Proceedings relating to the

---

* The word *object* requires explanation. Again and again it is used in the minutes and clearly in an entirely different sense from that in which we often use it today. To us, referring to a person as an 'object' usually implies that he looks ridiculous. In the eighteenth century 'an object' was someone about which something ought to be done, that generation talking about objects when we would talk about patients or cases, or refer to a person as deserving of charity or help.

Charity from the first Establishment thereof and how the Same had been conducted'. He told them that £600 had been received in the form of subscriptions and £40 collected out of the poor box; £100 had been spent on furniture, £32 on firing, £7 on candles, £69 on repairs, £34 on rent and taxes, £66 on wages, £146 on the dispensary, £3 on soap, £14 on stationery, and £17 on petty expenses, leaving £57 in hand. There were thirty patients in the house and three hundred on the books as out-patients. Of the 127 patients admitted during this period 10 had died, 12 had been discharged as incurable and 105 as cured. Two thousand had been treated as out-patients; of these, 93 were known to be dead and 49 had been discharged for misbehaviour or 'at their own Desire'. 815 had returned thanks for being cured but in the case of out-patients returning thanks was difficult to enforce: 876 had not bothered to conform but most were 'known to have been Cured'.

Getting the Duke of Richmond as president had certainly been a coup and an annual festival was inaugurated at John Harrison's suggestion, the idea of it being to keep the struggling infirmary in Prescott Street before the eyes of the public. '15th June 1742. On this day the Feast intended to be Anniversary was held for the first time at Mercers' Hall. Before dinner a Sermon was preached at Mercers' Chapple by the Revd Audley, Chaplain to the Infirmary, and a collection made at the Chapple doors for the benefit of the Charity. The Gentlemen then went to dinner at the Hall where an elegant Entertainment was provided for them by Ebeneezer Mussell, Esq., William Myre, Esq., and John Snee, Esq., as Stewards. After Dinner another collection was made among the Gentlemen present for the Benefit of the Charity and both collections amounted to £34-11-6. The Stewards' healths were drunk with Thanks to them for their handsome Entertainments.'

A major problem had been finding the right women to nurse the patients. The sisters of pre-Reformation days had disappeared at the dissolution. Nursing had not yet been rediscovered as a profession for women, and the committee had been compelled to recruit, without asking too many questions, elderly women, most of uncertain sobriety and doubtful past, who could no longer earn a living in other ways. The first mention of any such person as a nurse is when we read in the minutes 'that Squire be Contracted with by the Chairman of the Committee as a Nurse for the Women's ward at the rate of £14 a year'. The committee also engaged a night nurse, or 'watch' as night nurses were then called, at an annual salary of £9, the 'watches' at that date acknowledged to be of lower social standing than the day nurses. Soon others had to be engaged, and all were required to live in, their salaries reduced to £6 and £4 respectively in return for board and lodging. The duties of the day nurses were clearly defined: 'to enter upon their Business every morning at six in Summer, and at seven in Winter, to sup at ten and be in bed by eleven every Night; to clean their wards, pewter and utensils every day by seven in the morning; to attend the patients diligently during their Watch, and provide them with what is directed by the Physician, Surgeon and Apothecary, and see particularly that they take their medicines, and to keep the beds of the Patients neat and decent'. Finally, they were enjoined 'to behave with Tenderness to the Patients and with Curtesy and respect to Strangers'. Days off are not mentioned: holidays had not been invented.

Many proved unsuitable. Sarah Spencer 'was found to be lame in her left arm'; Mary Paul, 'guilty of mistakes in giving the Patients their Physick'. Some attempted to make money out of the patients: Squire did, but she was not dismissed, 'as it was not in the Rules that she should not do so', and Priscilla Banks, who 'sold bread and butter to the patients', was 'continued' on the 'insistence' of the Rev. Matthew Audley. The patients often complained about the nurses. Abraham Rim declared that he 'had 9/2 in his pocket, when received into the House and that Margaret Sparrow, the watch in John's Ward, did take his britches into her Room when she put him to bed and that in the morning he had missed his money'. In this case the committee discharged the watch and ordered the money to be deducted from her wages. But they did not always take the patient's side. When another complained that 'she had several times been refused Chicken, Rabit and Water Gruel, and had been called Bitch by Nurse

Squibb', they 'enquired into the Affair and found the Accusation untrue'.

Nurses who offended seriously were dismissed summarily. Nurse Lewin was discharged 'for Misbehaviour'; Susannah Woodbridge 'for Misdemeanour'; Phoebe Burnham for 'being disguised in liquor'. Nurse Stevens was found so drunk 'as to be unable to perform her Duties'. When two nurses 'prayed to be allowed some cordials', both were dismissed. For these were the days of Hogarth's *Gin Lane*; 'drunk for a penny, dead drunk for two pence'. One of the governors' main problems was to keep the household sober.

Nurses at that date were not all as bad as is painted. Lack of moral sense and insobriety were not incompatible with kindness of heart, and the service of the many who did their work well is occasionally recorded. The Westminster received a letter from 'the London' testifying to the excellent qualities of a nurse engaged after working there. It was possible, too, to get a patient 'specialed' even in those days. An 'extraordinary nurse' for a patient with smallpox got two shillings above her usual wage. A nurse was specially engaged to look after a child of five, admitted in spite of the regulation which stated that no children under six were to be taken into the house. Nor does the gratitude of the patients to the nurses pass unrecorded. Mary Kirby, who died in the infirmary, 'desired that her Cloathes might be divided among the Nurses and Watches, which was ordered accordingly, it being thought Reasonable that the Intention of the deceased should be Complied with'.

The first mention of a matron is when she was instructed 'to get a Firkin of Soap and bespeak some Candles'; this was Ann Looker, the wife of the porter. She did not last long. She was soon found guilty of 'bringing Spiritous Liquors into the House', and an advertisement for a new matron was inserted in the daily papers. Six applications were received and the candidates all interviewed at a special meeting of the court of governors. Thirty-five turned up and Mrs Broad was elected by ballot.

Now, that is to say after the infirmary had been open for about a year in Prescott Street, the committee decided to undertake the in-patient treatment of syphilis. (At that time this consisted of inunction of mercury which had the unfortunate side-effect of inducing copious salivation and often had to be pressed to the point at which it affected the jaw and began to loosen the teeth.) So another house farther down the street was taken to serve as a lock, as all hospitals for the treatment of syphilis were called in those days – the origin of the term is uncertain – at a rent of £10 per annum. Mrs Eliza Gilbert was appointed matron of it at £15 per annum but 'to provide herself with Diet at her own Charge'. Smallpox and cases of other contagious disease were also admitted to it, and before long the pressure on the beds in the infirmary was so great that the porter and general labourer had to share a bed in it. Nurses were even lodged there when there was no room for them elsewhere.

Within three years the work of the infirmary had in fact increased so much that when Dr John Cunningham offered his services he was elected physician extraordinary to help Dr Andrée.

William Petty, Master of the Barber Surgeons' Company, although already over seventy, also offered his services and was duly elected surgeon extraordinary. At this time joint rounds, something almost revolutionary in the history of the rivalry between physicians and surgeons, were started. 'Dr Andrée acquainted the Board that Agreeable to an Order of the last Committee he had with Dr Cunningham and the Surgeons agreed to meet every Wednesday precisely at 12 o'clock in order to visit the several Wards.'

Then John Harrison was taken ill and someone had to be found to do his work. Petty was considered too old, and the committee chose a certain Henry Dobson. The governors dug in their heels, however, and insisted on advertising the vacancy and on election by ballot. Many gentlemen, we are told, hurried to pay their subscriptions and so gain the right to vote for one of the four candidates who now applied. On the day of the election eighty-five governors turned up, seven ladies voted by proxy, and Dobson was elected after all, by a majority of forty-nine.

Within four years the demand for beds was so great that the

governors had been forced into renting the three houses adjacent to the infirmary. They paved the roadway outside and constructed steps up to the front door 'to make it easier for the Gentlemen to alight from their Chariots'. A row of posts with railings was erected in front of them, and two obelisks carrying oil lamps. On the 'fascia' of the four houses was inscribed in large letters:

THE LONDON INFIRMARY SUPPORTED BY
VOLUNTARY CONTRIBUTIONS
BEGUN NOV. 3, 1740

The annual festival of that year proved an outstanding success. A committee of eight stewards, appointed to make the arrangements, had held many meetings at a nearby tavern. Notices of it had been inserted in the press, five hundred tickets printed and a large number sent out to important people; a special invitation had been sent to the Lord Mayor and Sheriffs. The remaining tickets had been sold at 5s. and dinner ordered for two hundred and fifty, to be provided by Mr Davis 'according to his Bill of Fare delivered'.

After the sermon preached by the Bishop of Worcester, in which he had extolled the good work being done by the infirmary and launched an appeal for funds to build a new hospital when the present lease expired, John Harrison marshalled the procession to the Drapers' Hall. First came the beadles, provided with new uniforms for the occasion; then the president in his coach followed by the governors; then the physicians, the surgeons and lay staff bringing up the rear. The bells of St Lawrence rang out (for which the stewards paid £1. 10s.) as the procession left the church, and the bells of St Michael's, Cornhill (for which they paid £2. 2s.) as it passed. On arrival at the Drapers' Hall the company sat down to dinner at six tables, the top one dignified by silver candlesticks lent by Mr Fotherley Baker. (Many of the diners had brought their own servants to wait on them.) Claret, madeira and port were provided, and innumerable toasts were drunk. A French-horn blower had been engaged but whether to blow the procession through the City or entertain the company at dinner is not

clear. The latter had cost £103, of which £69 had been raised
out of the sale of tickets and the eight stewards between them, as
was understood, had stumped up the deficit on the evening's
work.

A considerable sum had been collected on behalf of the charity
both in church and at the dinner, but the real importance of the
occasion lay in the bishop's sermon. Isaac Maddox, born as
Aldersgate, educated at a charity school, and apprenticed to a
pastry cook, was certainly a friend of hospitals. Had he been the
first to see the necessity to build a new hospital – or was it John
Harrison again, and the bishop his mouthpiece? That we do
not know.

2

Growing Pains

Five years old! The infirmary, after six months' embryonic existence, as it can be aptly called, had been born into East London and now stood in the heart of a notoriously unsavoury area. Patronized by the nobility, it was maintained financially by the gentry and the fast-growing middle class.

The house committee, after the Mrs Looker affair, now took over the catering and entered into contract with various tradesmen: with Catersby & Holloway, brewers in Whitechapel, to provide ale and beer; with Mr Gordon to supply meat; with Enoch Alton for oatmeal. Every patient was allowed a 12 oz. loaf and meat on a scale which seems prodigious to modern standards. Further, if it was not considered up to standard, Mr Gordon was called before the committee and warned that he might lose his contract. The staff, or family as they were often termed, got the best cuts; the patients, 'the scragg and veiney Pieces'. The former got everything on a liberal scale: 'agreed that the Matron and Porter be allowed Diet at a rate of 2d loaf a day, 2 pounds of Beef or Mutton and double quantity of Butter and Cheese allowed each Patient'. Diet sheets, to which the nursing staff were required to adhere, were posted in every ward. When Mrs Broad reported that 'the allowance of Veal was too small to make the broth for Patients on the low Diet', the committee resolved 'that the Matron do make addition of so much scrag of mutton as may be necessary to better it and that, as some Patients cannot eat Milk

Potage, the Matron do make such alteration in their spoon meat as may be necessary'.

The governors also paid great attention to the spiritual welfare of the patients and, true to the habit of their day, tended to force religion down their throats. The Rev. Matthew Audley, rector of Rotherhithe, had offered his services to the infirmary soon after the move to Prescott Street – one pictures him being ferried across the river in a boat – and now read prayers in the committee room every Tuesday and performed the 'other necessary Duties of his Function'. He also preached a weekly sermon, attended by all members of the committee. On Sundays his obligations to his parish kept him away but, by order of the committee, a Bible and Book of Common Prayer were chained to a desk in each ward. When the Bishop of Bristol presented three dozen copies of *The Knowledge and Practice of Christianity made easy to the Meanest Capacities*, they ordered that one of these should also be chained to the desk in each ward for the benefit of patients.

As the work of the infirmary increased it became necessary to employ a secretary, and Richard Neale was appointed at a salary of 10 gns per annum. He was required 'to reside near the Infirmary; to write all Letters to Noblemen and others; to attend the House Visitors Twice a week; to collect Subscriptions; to enter the Patients' names in proper Books; to keep the Accounts and House Books; to Make out all Summonses; and also to do all the other Business where writing is required in the two Houses'. Later, when his recording proved inaccurate, he was required to write up the minutes of every meeting before leaving the room.

The drugs ordered by the physicians had to be supplied and new items bought from time to time to equip the 'elaboratory': among others, 'a pewter Crane and Mulligator' and 'a levigating Stone'. (To levigate was to reduce to a fine powder.) Then, when Mr Cole retired, Godfrey Webb was elected to replace him. He was a young man and the terms on which he was appointed strict: to put down £100 to cover the charity against the risk of his dishonesty; to furnish his own room and 'to provide himself with his own Diet and Washing'. Nor was he ever to be absent without leave or when the physicians and surgeons were doing their rounds. When he did go out, he was required 'to leave in the Key hole of the Apothecary's room a note specifying the Place to which he had gone that in case of any Emergency he may be sent for'. Nor was he ever 'to lye abroad or be absent from the House after 10 o'clock at Night, or to bring any Wife or Child into the House that he may now have or may hereafter have under any Pretext whatever'.

His professional duties were also made clear. He was to maintain 'a sufficient quantity of Pills, Powders, Electuaries and other Preparations ready to be delivered to the Patients' and to keep a written record of all drugs coming into and going out of the dispensary. A committee of 'Physical Gentlemen that are Subscribers' was appointed to audit his books and 'such Governors as were skilled in Pharmacy and Drugs' were asked to inspect and report on his medicines from time to time. Finally, before taking up his office, he was required to swear that 'he would faithfully Prepare and Dispense medicines to the best of his Ability and Judgement', and 'not Imbezzle any of them or put them to any other Use but what they are or shall be really Designed for'.

As time went on the committee seems to have relented towards him. He was provided with his meals in the house, apparently dining in solitary state. His 'Cloath was now to be laid where he shall think Proper, and the Provisions for the family Dinner brought up to him to take what he likes, then to be sent down to the Matron who shall sit at the head of the Table below stairs along with the Nurses, Watches, Messenger and assistant to the Elaboratory'. Before long, too, when he asked for help, Peter Grimes was engaged 'to assist in the Dispensary, and also keep the Garden in good and decent Order', and when Grimes became porter and messenger (in succession to Mr Looker), Wells Brandon was appointed in his place. (He was required to sleep 'under the counter in the dispensary in a feather Bed with Doors'.) Again and again this man caused trouble. Twice he is recorded as having been 'disguised in Liquor', and later the minutes relate how 'the Apothecary's man and the Cookmaid were Quarrelsome and given to Fighting to the Disturbance of the whole House'; and how eventually he was discharged 'for having struck the Cook-maid as evidenced by the other Servants'. Nor was his successor a success. 'Joseph Watts, who pounds in the Mortar, being reported as addicted to Drinking and being on his examination much disguised in Liquor, was ordered to be immediately Discharged.'

Then further trouble: Peter Grimes, porter and messenger, absconded with various items of hospital property and cashed in on his connection with the infirmary by getting a job as a ship's surgeon's mate. This infuriated 'the gentlemen of the committee' who now passed an order to the effect that 'Peter Grimes be immediately discharged' – he had long since taken himself off – and 'cautioned not to make Pretence of having been taught Surgery here'.

The committee now took the opportunity to replace the porter-messenger by 'two persons under the denomination of upper and lower Beadle'. They were provided with 'lodging and diet, and livery Coat and Frock to be worn on the service of the Charity only'. The upper was 'to carry all Letters that relate to the Charity, and to attend the Surgery and all Meetings of the Governors'; the lower to attend the physicians and apothecary and act as pounder to the elaboratory man. The committee set great store on their appearance as likely to impress the governors who came to courts at the infirmary. 'Agreed that their Liveries be made of blue Cloath with red Button Holes and a scarlet Waistcoat and in the room of cloath to have blue shagg Breeches.' It was terribly important, too, to have them looking smart at the annual festival. 'Ordered that the Beadles have new Liveries, new Gowns, and new great Coats against the Feast day, the new gowns to be worn only on the Feast Day and on the days of General Courts and their old Gowns on Committee days.' In spite of this they caused trouble too. 'A complaint being made by Mary Everett, late an in-patient in Rachel's ward, against Ephraim Shore and John Cushee for coming into the Ward on Xmas night at an unreasonable Time after the Patients were in bed, and for the said Shore swearing and behaving indecently and playing and dallying with one of the patients for a considerable Time, Agreed that the said Shore be immediately discharged.' Cushee was 'continued' and eventually made good. 'A motion being made that John Cushee shall have some Gratuity for his extraordinary Trouble on his duty in the House', the steward was instructed to pay him two guineas out of petty cash.

A new matron now had to be found for the lock as Mrs Gilbert had been allowed to go off and look after her father and had not returned, so the post was advertised in the press. This produced three petitioners, or candidates as we would call them, who were interviewed by the whole court of governors. Nearly a hundred turned up and Mrs Gouy, about whom we shall hear more, was elected by 50 votes to 42 over Mrs Hind. At the same meeting it was agreed to take over the house next door so as to enlarge the lock. They also publicized in the *Daily Advertiser* their readiness to treat venereal disease. These patients, presumably on account of the social stigma attached to it, were handled differently from all the rest. Out-patients were required to deposit 10s. 6d. as a security against bad behaviour, to be refunded 'on returning Thanks'; in-patients to contribute 11s. 6d. a week towards their 'Subsistence during their Cure'.

The demand for more beds now steadily increased and any room that could be spared was incorporated into one of the wards. The steward was turned out of his and required to sleep in the committee room, the two beadles in the corridor and the apothecary in the physicians' room. Then the committee started to open beds in the lock, in spite of the recent decision, for purposes for which it had never been intended. The pressure on the general beds had become too great. 'Agreed that the Title upon the Fascia be taken down, other Persons being admitted therein besides those whose Cases required salivating.' Before long, too, so many 'extraordinary' and 'accidental' cases were being admitted that it even became necessary to put more than one patient in the same bed. 'Ordered that Mr Phipps do provide six pairs of large Blankets for the use of those Beds into which Matron is obliged to put two Patients.'

The problem of finding space for other purposes was also pressing. The governors were particularly worried because the infirmary had no chapel, in an age when listening to sermons was counted as essential to salvation. All sorts of benefits, too, were now believed to accrue from exposure of the body to cold water and those who could afford it had a cold bath installed in their own houses – something akin to the modern swimming pool. So John Harrison 'was desired to wait on Capt. Johnson and ask his leave to make use of his Cold Bath and, in case of Refusal, to make the best Bargain he could for such of their Patients in the House whose case required such Relief'. We do not know the results of this interview, or where Captain Johnson lived, but it was presumably unsuccessful as we now find the physicians demanding a cold bath of their own. They were also demanding a post-mortem room and the apothecary a 'levigating room' as an annexe to the 'elaboratory'. Nor was there yet any waiting-room for out-patients. These crowded the corridors to overflowing and, when the committee had attempted to solve this problem by converting a shed in the garden to this purpose, it had proved far from satisfactory; pots of ale were handed in through the window, we are told. So, when Mr Yond, the owner of a house near by, offered his ground floor as a waiting-room, the committee jumped at the offer as a temporary expedient.

The obvious solution of the whole problem was to build, and Mr Myre was asked to wait on Mr Leman, the landlord of the infirmary premises, 'to desire that a further conditional Term might be added to the present Lease of 21 years in consideration of the Building proposed in the room of the back Premises'. Mr Myre was a personal friend of Mr Leman's and had been chosen for this mission on that account. But he failed: he was obliged to report to the committee that, although he had 'urged the Affair as much as possible, Mr Leman absolutely declined to grant any optional Terms'.

In spite of this rebuff the governors decided to go ahead with their building. This, when finished, provided a chapel, a cold bath, a waiting-room for out-patients and a dead-house above which a room was set apart 'for opening the bodies of such extraordinary Bodies as are directed by the Physicians'. But it had cost the committee much more than they had reckoned. The wall separating the infirmary from Mr Yond's house, the same Mr

Yond as had offered his ground floor as a waiting-room, had had to be rebuilt because he threatened legal proceedings unless they kept infirmary patients off his premises. The cold bath had caused trouble, too, as it kept on leaking. The governors had, however, increased the capital value of their leasehold property and now insured it for £2000 at an annual premium of £12 at the Hand in Hand fire office in Snow Hill.

The infirmary now maintained a hundred and thirty beds. Party walls had been pulled down and rooms thrown into one another to make the wards, referred to in the minutes as Martha's, Cole's, Vernon's, Fowler's, presumably the names of the nurses who looked after them. (Not until 1754 do we read of Richmond, so called after the first president.) Their walls were covered with layers of old paper, and their floors with sand which the servants were required to sweep up every day and sift back on to them.

Medical treatment was mainly theoretical and correspondingly expensive. A committee of inquiry found that the drug bill for a year round about this date amounted to £580 of which £200 had been paid for malt spirit 'there being above 700 gallons used, making 2 gallons a day'. The rest had gone on elixirs, decoctions and other complicated medicines which the physician prescribed. Odd things, too, were sometimes used. Mary James, for instance, was paid 'one guinea for levigating eight pounds of Crabbes claws'. Blood letting, purgation, sweating, were the great stand-bys but the governors did not capitulate to any form of quackery that came along. When Mr John MacCape, surgeon and apothecary, 'acquainted them that by Experience he had found a nostrum for curing the Cancer without a Knife, and offering to use it for the relief of such poor Objects as may be in the Hospital under that dreadful disorder', they saw through him. They thought it altogether improper 'to allow him the Liberty he desired, or to suffer that any experiments be made upon the Patients of the Hospital'.

Surgery, on the other hand, was based on sound principles and even in pre-anaesthetic and pre-Listerian days surgeons got good results in spite of the fact that healing 'by first intention' was rare;

B

infection and suppuration were almost inevitable. Repeated dressing of most wounds was necessary, with the result that one of the
many problems of the committee was to keep the surgeons
adequately supplied with lint. This was made by scraping cotton
or flaxen fabric with a semi-sharp instrument which broke up its
threads and raised a rough woolly surface. So important, in fact,
was lint, and so slow its production, that a lint-scraper was paid
more than a nurse – paid, too, by the quarter, her salary always
kept a quarter in arrear in case she did not produce enough and to
stop her absconding. Other women took on lint making as piece-
work. 'Agreed that Mary Manser, Mary Rose, and Ann Looker
[the former matron] be employed to scrape lint for the use of the
Surgeons, to be furnished with Cloaths for that purpose by the
Matron, and that Mary Manser be allowed $\frac{1}{2}$ crown a pound and
her Board in the Lock.'

The mortality of compound fractures was exceptionally high,
only fifty per cent or so surviving to require artificial limbs. These
were very expensive. Early in the history of the infirmary the
minutes record that an iron was to be made 'for Mr Harley
to be returned when done with'; a little later that Susan Smith
was 'to be allowed a wooden leg'. A national fund was started for
the benefit of the wounded 'in the late rebellion' (of 1745), and
the charity, 'as it had received so many Objects as were sufferers
in it', was awarded £100. As time went on, artificial limbs
became more efficient although at the same time more expensive
still, and as late as 1757 'it was not customary to give wooden legs
except in cases of great Poverty and Distress'. Under this saving
clause some qualified for them. On one occasion the steward 'was
ordered to pay the following sums out of the petty cash account,
viz. an Arm above the elbow with steel plate and hooks for Anne
Jones 10s., and 7s. for a leg below the knee with balls and cushion
for Thomas Lant'.

Many distempers – as diseases were then called – were clearly
infectious, transmitted from man to man, and the committee
strove to keep them out of the house in so far as that was possible
when the way in which they spread was not understood. 'No
Persons suspected of having the Small Pox, itch or any other

infectious or venereal Distemper or judged to have a Consumptive condition' were to be admitted 'on any account whatever.' Arrangements were made with the Smallpox Hospital 'to receive any such sick Persons under this Complaint as shall be recommended by this Charity'. The committee subscribed five guineas to it in the name of John Harrison. Two years later it increased this to ten, 'the number of Objects sent to the Small Pox Hospital having exceeded that Number apprehended', but every now and then the committee got landed with a case. 'Ordered that Thomas Cook, recommended by Mr William Martin, having the Smallpox full on him and immediate Assistance necessary, be provided with a Lodging at hand and taken care of at the Expense of the Infirmary, and that Mr Martin be acquainted that the Committee were surprised at his sending an Object so contrary to the rules of this Charity.'

The committee also continued to refuse to admit pregnant women, but on at least one occasion a woman at or near full term succeeded in getting past them. 'Elizabeth Brazier, having been delivered of a female child in the House on Thursday morning, Ordered, as its father could not be found, that the said child be sent to the Foundling Hospital immediately.' They also continued to refuse children under seven except those with fractures or requiring amputations and those with exceptional conditions. 'Agreed that James Levison, a child of five years, be received into the Infirmary to be cut for the Stone.' Nor did they accept 'persons disordered in their Senses'. Mental patients were packed off to Bethlem but these, like pregnant women, sometimes got past the committee's defences. 'Elizabeth Cracraft, an in-patient recommended by Mr David Barclay, being found a Lunatick, the Secretary was ordered to acquaint Mr Barclay thereof and desire him to order her to be removed.' Malingerers and hysterics, too, often succeeded in getting in. 'Ordered that Garrard Brown be discharged, it appearing from the Report of the Surgeons that there is no foundation for his Complaint.'

Epileptics often caused disturbances in the wards. 'It having been found by daily Experience that Patients troubled with Fits are a cause of a great deal of Inconvenience in the House, not only by frightening into the same Distemper some who were never subject to it before, but also by frequently occasioning a Relapse to such as were almost cured, and as they can be treated as out-patients, Ordered that they be treated as such.'

The committee also had to guard against blocking the beds with patients for whom they could do nothing. Early in the history of the infirmary a regulation had been made against admitting any in a 'dieing condition'. Now they were compelled to legislate against filling up the beds with chronics. 'Ordered that no Patient deemed incurable or in a consumptive or asthmatical Condition, being more capable of Relief as out-patients, or any Person having an ulcer of long standing, be admitted into the House.' Varicose ulcers, then as now, were common. 'Mr Dodson having informed the Committee that a great number of women Patients had been cured of ulcerated Legs, but some short time afterwards the Ulcers have broken out again, which is occasioned by their not wearing proper bandages, Recommended that a pattern be bought for each of your Matrons of laced Stockings, knee pieces and ankle pieces, so that the same sort may be made by such patients and given them when discharged.'

The lay members of the committee continued to play an active part in deciding which of 'the poor Objects' sent up by the governors should be admitted, but the decision in respect of 'accidental' cases often had to rest on other shoulders. Sometimes it seems to have been expected of the matrons or even of a nurse. Elizabeth Ayers, nurse Richmond, and Mary Gouy, now assistant matron to Mrs Broad, for instance, were held responsible for refusing to admit James Chapman, brought up with a fractured skull. This offence, said the committee, demanded 'instant dismissal' but, as it was Mrs Gouy's first, they agreed 'to accept her Submission and promise of better behaviour in the future'.

In these days it would have been left at that; indeed every effort would be made to cover up a mistake of that kind. Not so in the eighteenth century: 'Sensable of how much an Affair of this kind may Injure the Charity in the Opinion of the world', the committee insisted on 'a signed recantation' to be published in the newspapers:

> *London Hospital, 12 Mar. 1745.*
>
> *Whereas I, Mary Gouy, one of the Matrons of this Charity, have been guilty of a Notorious breach of my Duty in Acting in direct Opposition of one of the known Laws relative to my Office, viz. That I am to receive accidents at all hours, and Immediately acquaint the Physicians and Surgeons, and instead of so doing I did as far as in me lay refuse Admittance into this Hospital, James Chapman, sent in as an Accident for a fractured skull on the 7th instant, by telling his Friends who brought him hither about Seven oClock in the Evening that it was an Improper hour, and that he must be brought again the next morning at Eleven oClock by which delay the Patient in the opinion of the Surgeons might Suffer and his cure be retarded, I do hereby humbly acknowledge my Fault, and promise never again to be guilty of the same, and being truly sensable how greatly this Behaviour of mine in the Opinion of the World may injure the Charity, whose invariable Rule it has always been to Admit all Accidents whether Recommended or not, at all hours of the day or night, do Take this publick method of acknowledging my Fault, and the great Laxity of the House Committee in Receiving me back into their favour, on my Sincere promise of never offending in the like or any other manner* whatsoever *for the Future. Mary Gouy.*

The beds were bare wood at first but now upholstered, and the committee also reported, with a touch of pride, that there was now 'a pair of Sheets to each Bed'! Oilcloths had also been bought for four of them for the benefit of 'Patients incapable of keeping themselves clean', and 'three sets of Apparel for men and the same number for women Patients whose necessities render them Naked at their admission or who from the Vermin or other causes might make it necessary for them to change their Cloathes for a time'. Cross-infection of a gastro-intestinal kind frequently complicated the nursing problem. 'Among the Objects received into the Charity some of them afterwards become affected with Distempers which render them Obnoxious to the other Patients and there being a vacant room, your Committee directed three

Beds be made for the Reception of such Objects whose particular cases render them offensive.'

There were no sinks in the house. 'Complaints having been made that the Servants throw out the Wastwater into Prescott Street at any time most convenient to themselves, which is very Offensive to all the neighbours, your Committee has ordered for the Future that such Wastwater may be thrown out into the Kennel before the doors, and that the Pavement be properly mended for such water to run off.' Nor did sanitation, as we conceive it, yet exist. There was no water flushing, and no drains except for surface water. So 'the soil', which had accumulated during the day in the ward privies and close-stools, had to be carried down in buckets and dumped in the street for the nightman to cart away. 'Mr James May, the Nightman, attended this day and informed the Committee that the men employed to carry away the soil from the necessary House had also carried away 15 tons out of the cesspool belonging to Mrs Gouy's Kitchen.' And again, later: 'Ordered that the Chairman do draw on the Treasurer to James Brand, the Nightman, for £15. 8s. 0d. for carrying away 72 loads of Soil from the necessary House, together with 12s. for candles and beer to his servants.'

The cesspools also had to be pumped out at intervals. 'Whereas Complaints have been made that the Pumping the Sullidge water from the several Cesspools belonging to this Hospital into Chamber Street [behind the hospital parallel with Prescott Street] is so offensive to the Inhabitants that they cannot live in their Houses, and several of them threatening Bills of Inditement against us if the same be continued, Mr Mainwaring [who had recently been appointed surveyor] advised digging a cesspool in the middle of the Garden down to the Springs which would carry off the Sullidge water and prevent Pumping.' This idea did not work. Pumping into Chamber Street had to be continued and again and again the local residents would take direct action to try to stop it. 'Ordered that when the Labourer is obliged to pump the Sullidge water, the two Beadles do attend alternately to prevent any Person stopping the Pipe up.'

The atmosphere of the wards must have been dreadful; pots

of aromatic herbs were put in all of them in a vain attempt to improve it. A better plan would have been to keep the windows open, but the attitude of the medical profession to fresh air at that date was curious: 'Ordered that the Windows be not opened or left open especially in the Evenings without leave of the Physicians or Surgeons or in their absence of the Apothecary.' There may also have been sound reasons for this: 'the poor Patients in danger of catching Cold for want of Covering'. In due course some change took place in the attitude of the profession: 'Ordered that the Windows be opened at the Top for the Convenience of the Patients.'

Epidemics of infection of a gastro-intestinal kind were common and bedclothes must often have got into a shocking state. 'Great Inconvenience', we are also told, 'arose from the beds not being aired and cleansed after the removal or death of the Patients, another often being directly put into it.' They also feared that a dirty bed might retain 'some part of the malignity of the distemper' of its previous occupant. So they now advertised for a number of new beds 'the covering to be of substantial British ticking and the filling of the best sweet Flocks from woolen cloth Rags'. These were supplied by William Petty of Rotherhithe at 16s. each. There are no references to the nurses washing the patients; that they washed, or were washed much, seems unlikely. In 1748 'the Consideration of having a hot bathing Tub' was postponed *sine die*, and there is no mention of any such thing again until four years later when it was agreed 'that a bathing Tub $2\frac{1}{2}$ feet high be provided at the desire of Dr Stibbins'.

The physicians and surgeons now recommended 'a common diet for those in the House'. Pudding, nature unspecified, now replaced meat three days a week; the other main items were milk potage, water gruel, rice milk and butter or cheese. Fresh vegetables seem to us a strange omission but turnips are mentioned, and large quantities of lemon and, later, lime juice, on the relative merits of which the physicians were asked to pronounce, were used in the dispensary. What for is not clear, as this certainly started before James Long published his *Treatise on the Scurvey* in 1753.

Small beer remained the standard drink and was liberally supplied; the fact that every quarter about thirty shillings, derived from the sale of yeast, was handed over by the matrons suggests that it was brewed on the premises. Tea was still an expensive commodity and regarded by Jonas Hanway, a governor and eighteenth-century eccentric, as 'destructive of public morals'. Anyhow, for either moral or financial reasons, the committee took the view that tea drinking must be controlled. When nurse Grubs and Anne Hound, a patient, were reported drinking tea at eleven o'clock at night, they were reprimanded. Later, on hearing 'that Tea is *frequently* drunk in the Wards among the Patients to entertain the Nurses and Watches', the committee considered prohibiting it altogether. Eventually they compromised. 'Ordered that for the Future no patient in the Hospital shall drink any Tea without the Permission of one of the Physicians or Surgeons or the Apothecary or of one of the Matrons of the House.'

By 1746 further additions to the staff had become necessary. James Stibbins (who insisted on the wash tub) was elected assistant physician; Walter Jones, assistant surgeon. John Harrison continued to do most of the surgical work and now asked for a furnished room 'for lying in, alleging it to be for the Safety of Patients in capital Operations to be immediately at Hand'. His health was beginning to fail, however, and other arrangements soon had to be made, the surgeons representing to the committee 'that it was Necessary for one of their Pupils to be resident at the Infirmary to be ready for any accidents or emergencies that may happen, several Inconveniences having been found for want of such Assistance'. So Harrison offered his own pupil and it was agreed that he 'should have his board with Mrs Gouy and lodge in Mr Harrison's apartment'.

Three years later Dr Cunningham died and the governors decided to advertise the vacancy in all the leading papers and elect by ballot. This was to start at 11 a.m. and close at 2 p.m. A thousand balloting papers were printed and the committee room got ready, the barrier which normally separated its members from the patients at their weekly meetings being taken down, the floor matted, and the doors, we are told, made warm 'for the reception of the Governors'. At 10 a.m. on the day appointed, fifty had turned up and the three candidates were called in, and their petitions (to be elected) read, followed by the letters of the noblemen and ladies who were sending proxies to vote on their behalf. Then the ballot started. By 2 p.m. 363 votes had been cast and Dr Sylvester, an M.D. of Leyden, had been elected by a majority of 121.

Looking back now, the crowd of governors that flocked to the little house which constituted the infirmary for this and subsequent elections of its kind, and the number of noblemen and ladies who bothered to send proxies to vote on their behalf, seem quite extraordinary. Certainly it is difficult to believe either that more than a handful of them possessed any real knowledge of the relative merits of the candidates or were seriously concerned about getting the right man in. Rather, the explanation would seem to lie in the complex system of patronage which dominated eighteenth-century society. It paid the middle class to work under aristocratic patrons and always vote as they did on all issues; paid the upper class, too, to patronize and to have votes on which they could rely. Candidates who secured a patron could be sure of the votes of all his satellites, and it was the candidates who secured the most influential patrons who usually got elected. Thus the nobility governed the hospital and, in spite of what one may feel about the system today, usually governed it well.

The extent of aristocratic patronage of the little infirmary tucked away in Goodmans Fields also seems extraordinary. The Dukes of Richmond, Devonshire and Bedford, the two archbishops, many bishops, the Lord Chancellor, the Master of the Rolls, the Lord Chief Justice and the Baron of the Exchequer had all been persuaded into becoming life governors. How had that come about? Almost certainly through the influence of the president, the Duke of Richmond, who had been persuaded to take an interest in the charity by John Harrison from its beginning and had become its first president. A Whig and an ardent supporter of the Hanoverian succession he had been with the King at Dettingen and served with the Duke of Cumberland at Culloden. He was much in royal favour. There is, indeed, good reason to suppose

that it was 'the London's' first president who gained the interest
in it of the great officers of state, and of so many of the temporal
and spiritual peers, and also laid the foundation of its future
association with the royal family.

Meanwhile the annual festival was on a bigger scale than ever,
although always following the same general pattern – the bishop's
sermon, the procession, the dinner at the city hall – and it continued to keep the charity in Goodmans Fields before the eyes of
the public. The beadles decked out in their new livery headed the
procession. Trumpeters were engaged and the City Marshal
called in to organize it. (In previous years some outsiders had
managed to join the procession and gatecrashed the party, so
the apothecary and steward were now stationed at the door to
check the gentlemen's tickets.) After these occasions, too, the
bishop's sermon was printed with the balance sheet and a report
on the work of the charity during the past year. These, together
with subscription and legacy forms, were widely circulated and
constituted, as it would be called later, an appeal on behalf of the
charity.

Each year, with the festival in full swing, the daily routine of
the infirmary had to be carried on and those left on duty were not
forgotten. 'Ordered that the Matron provide 2 hams not exceeding 16 lbs. each and 2 joints of veal, twelve bottles of Wine and
12 quarts of Porter for themselves and the Servants of the House
on Feast day.'

3

Teenage Troubles

The hospital in its early teens – *hospital* was gradually replacing *infirmary* in all references to it – was now overtaken by two misfortunes both of which might have been attended by serious consequences to an institution depending for its continued existence entirely on voluntary contribution.

The first was bred of individual dishonesty. Members of the committee noticed that the secretary, Richard Neale, did not always hand in the infirmary books in the evenings and that the minutes of meetings were not being kept up to date. Before long their suspicions were aroused in other directions and a sub-committee appointed to scrutinize the infirmary accounts for the last nine years. This soon revealed that nearly five hundred pounds – a lot of money in those days – received as subscriptions had never been brought into them. Neale might have been sacked outright but inquiry revealed that he had got into serious domestic difficulties, and he was merely suspended. Sir Samuel Cox, one of the governors, partly out of compassion for Neale and partly to avoid open scandal, persuaded eight other governors to join with him to replace the money, and the interest on it, within two years. Neale was now reinstated in his office by the unanimous vote of the governors. He must have had good points. But, less than a year later, overcome by the disgrace or overtaken by further domestic troubles – which of these is not clear – he resigned and took himself off.

A new secretary now had to be appointed and Gifford, the

house steward, and three others offered themselves. The governors took no chances this time. The successful candidate was to be required to put down £500 to cover them against his possible dishonesty, to live in and never 'to lie out of the House after 11 o'clock at night at the farthest'. Again the election was by ballot of the whole court and the turn-out of governors remarkable. Three hundred and forty arrived to vote and sixteen noblemen and ladies sent proxies. By 3 p.m. Mr Trotter had defeated Mr Gifford by a majority of twenty-two.

The second misfortune which overtook the charity was bred of professional rivalry. The infirmary was no longer quite the same happy place as it had been in its early days. New members of the medical staff had been elected and a flaming row now broke out between the physicians and the surgeons. The former started it. 'The many Inconveniences,' they wrote to the committee, 'which arise daily from the Provinces of Physick and Surgery being unsettled and undetermined in this Hospital oblige us to beg you to report to the next General Court the Necessity of a Special Committee in order to fix and determine the Practice of Physick and Surgery in the House which will obviate the many occasions of Dispute which daily occur and greatly contribute to the welfare of the patients and the honour of the Hospital.'

On receipt of this communication, the committee asked the physicians for their 'propositions'. These amounted to nothing less than that the surgeons were to be forbidden to prescribe any drugs of any kind by the mouth (internals) except purgatives. This, of course, seems absurd to us now, but medicine (or physick, as it was then called) and surgery had originated in very different ways; the former as the result of theory elaborated in the universities; the latter in consequence of practical experience gained on the battlefield and in the barbers' shop. The Royal College of Physicians and Surgeons' Hall guarded their respective privileges jealously.

The house committee, faced with this situation, called a special meeting to which both parties to the dispute were summoned. First they listened to what the physicians had to say and 'to their Reasons for this Restriction'; then 'to the Objections of the

Surgeons'; then 'to the reply of the Physicians'. Both parties were then required to withdraw and the committee, 'having considered the arguments', and caring little about the privileges of the Royal College of Physicians, came down heavily on the side of the surgeons. It was agreed *nem con* 'that the present practice of Physick and Surgery in the Hospital be continued'. The surgeons were to continue to prescribe just as they thought fit.

This was more than their medical colleagues could stand, for it undermined both the dignity of their college and the whole concept of physick on which their reputation stood. So, understandably perhaps, they blundered. They drafted a petition to the president of the hospital behind the backs of the governors (who had accepted the verdict of their committee), expecting them, apparently, to reverse what was now a decision of the governors and come down on their side. Almost more stupidly, when the committee asked to see the petition, the physicians flatly refused. The house committee now lost their heads. 'Resolved that the late attempt of the Physicians on the Dignity and Power of the General Court and the Liberty of every Governor endangering likewise the Harmony that had always existed between the late President and their Hospital, appears to this Committee to be of such dangerous Consequences that they think it necessary to recommend to the next General Court to take such Steps as may effectively prevent any such mischievous Practices for the future.'

Second thoughts and wiser counsels soon prevailed. At their next meeting the committee rescinded this violent resolution and accepted a compromise – face-saving as far as the physicians were concerned – concocted by Shute Adams and Fotherley Baker the lawyer. The surgeons were to continue to prescribe 'internals' for their patients as they saw fit but 'on appearance of Danger' a physician was to be called in. It was also suggested – a suggestion which, as we have seen, had been made before but probably never acted upon – that the physicians and surgeons should go round the wards together 'to divide the Patients between them and see such as do require their mutual Assistance'.

The physicians accepted this compromise and apologized.

'Agreed to accept the Acknowledgement made by the Physicians', run the minutes of the governors, 'concerning their Behaviour to the House Committee and their presenting a Memorial to His Grace the late Duke of Richmond, as a full Satisfaction', cautioning them however against 'ever making any Complaint whatsoever for the Future relating to the Hospital except First to the House Committee and then to a General Court'. They went out of their way, too, to record that 'John Harrison, the Surgeon-in-Ordinary, had acquitted himself to the Satisfaction of the Committee in point of Practice on the Patients and had discharged his Duty in every respect as a surgeon to the Hospital'. Indeed, it looks much as if the behaviour of the physicians had been largely inspired by animosity against him. Perhaps it was Harrison who had been trespassing on their territory by prescribing drugs too freely.

This dispute had long-term consequences. Never again was a physician or surgeon elected to the staff allowed to serve as a governor. Further, the affairs of the charity were conducted so much in public that it might have had most damaging consequences. Many subscribers had already withdrawn their subscriptions. So the secretary was instructed to write round, telling them all that the 'late differences in the Hospital are now happily Adjusted' and begging 'the Continuance of their subscriptions to the Charity'.

The storm blew over and the physicians and surgeons began to work more together, but complaints against the hospital from time to time were inevitable and the committee, ever jealous of its reputation, endeavoured in every case to ascertain the facts and refute them, if they could. Mrs Parsons, for instance, who kept the ale house in Prescott Street, complained that William Farrell, scalded at her brewhouse near the hospital, had been ordered to return thanks in spite of the fact that he had never been properly cured. The committee went into the case. The surgeon said that he had been completely cured but 'had gone away with the crutches and cloathes that belong to the Hospital'. Mrs Parsons apologized. Shortly after this Mrs Hilton, a troublesome governor, told the committee that a patient in whom she was interested had been admitted with a compound fracture but had received no attention for three whole days! Again the committee found no truth in the man's story. So they waited on her in person and informed her of the facts, whereupon she withdrew her accusation and admitted that she must have been mistaken.

'I am credibly informed,' wrote the Bishop of Oxford, 'that Francis Flight, whom I lately recommended to you, was put into a Noiseome room and very ill Accommodated. I therefore desire proper Information concerning the true State of the Case, and that if any Fault or Neglect has happened, it may be Rectified.' An accusation from such an important person put the committee in a flutter and, after making the necessary inquiries, the secretary was instructed to reply to his lordship as follows:

> *The Man was layed in the Salivating ward, he being himself so Dirty and Offensive that he could not properly lay near anyone else. The Room is on the top of the House very low built and during the Winter has been so blacked with lamps as to have an indifferent Appearance tho warm and otherwise Convenient. Everything has been done for him that is Necessary towards his Cure and the Governors beg leave to acquaint Your Lordship that nothing shall be wanting in them for the Future tho in the fracture of the joint of a hip in a man so advanced in years they are very dubious of success.*

A little later John Hoylock, who had injured his hand with a pick and refused amputation, which the surgeon had advised, discharged himself and put himself under a surgeon at Stratford. The committee thought they had done all they could for him, and had no doubt forgotten all about him, until they heard not only that he had died but, to their dismay, that 'a scandalous attack' was circulating on the reputation of the hospital and on the 'tenderness, care and judgement of the surgeon'. He was 'starved', it was being said, 'while in the House and Neglected to be dressed for 3 days, and on his Declaring that he would not have his Arm taken off, Mr Harrison had told him that he might go and be damned'. Again the committee hastened to ascertain the facts. They 'inquired minutely into the affair of the Patients in the ward where he was placed', and were informed 'by John Comyn and James Neal who laid in the next Bed to him that the said John Hoylock never made any complaint of want of Diet, nor was there any room for him so to do, that he had been constantly attended and dressed and never heard any ill Language made use of by Mr Harrison, but on the contrary treated him with the greatest Tenderness and frequently endeavoured to persuade him to submit to what the Physicians and Surgeons advised'.

Complaints against John Harrison – by whom is never clear – eventually came to a head. 'The Committee, being informed that a Report was industriously spread that an Alteration was necessary to be made in the present Establishment of the Surgeons, thought it was their Duty to lay the same before the General Court but cannot but observe that they are well satisfied by the care taken by Mr Harrison, the Surgeon-in-Ordinary, of his Patients, not having any complaint of Neglect brought before them.' Mr Nettleton, however, one of the governors, pressed for an inquiry into 'the Practice and Management and Conduct of all the Officers and Servants of the Hospital'. So a special committee of inquiry was appointed under the chairmanship of John Gore, Esq., vice-president. Three months later they submitted a long report which throws much light on the organization of the hospital at that date.

'The Physicians', they found, 'attend regularly on the days prescribed for them, except on Sundays, when they only came if sent for.' This arrangement, the committee thought, might be prejudicial, particularly to patients suffering from fevers for whom prescriptions were often altered at frequent intervals. So they inquired into what was done in this matter. A physician, they were told, after visiting his own patients, would visit any other patient he was asked to see. The physicians in fact worked together and, if at any time no physician was available, 'the skill of the apothecary, and his knowledge of the methods practiced by the several Physicians', qualified him in their opinion to take full responsibility.

The surgeon-in-ordinary, Mr John Harrison, attended every day, except Sundays when in summer he was often out of town,

At a Meeting of the Subscribers to the intended
Infirmary had at the Feathers Tavern Cheapside
23d. September 1740
Present

Mr. John Snee Son.   Mr. John Harrison
Mr. Sclater   Mr. Josiah Cole
Mr. Fotherley Baker   Mr. Shute Adams
Mr. G. Potter

It was proposed and agreed to have a weekly Meeting And the
first to be on Tuesday the 29th Instant

Mr. Harrison delivered in the Lease of the House taken for the
intended Infirmary which was approv'd & returned to him to
keep the same till further Order of the Subscribers

Mr. Sclater was chosen Chairman for next Meeting to be held
at this Place at 7 oClock in the Evening

It was proposed that the several Subscriptions made to
compleat the Sum of 100 Guineas be produced next Tuesday the
30th Instant

A Motion was made, Whether with the Sum already subscrib.
it would be proper to begin the said Charity And unanimously
agreed it was

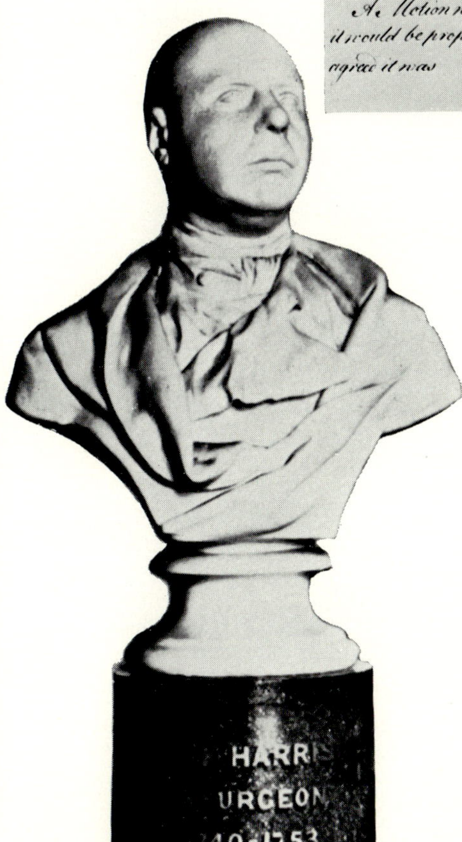

JOHN HARRISON, SURGEON
The bust by Robert Phipps

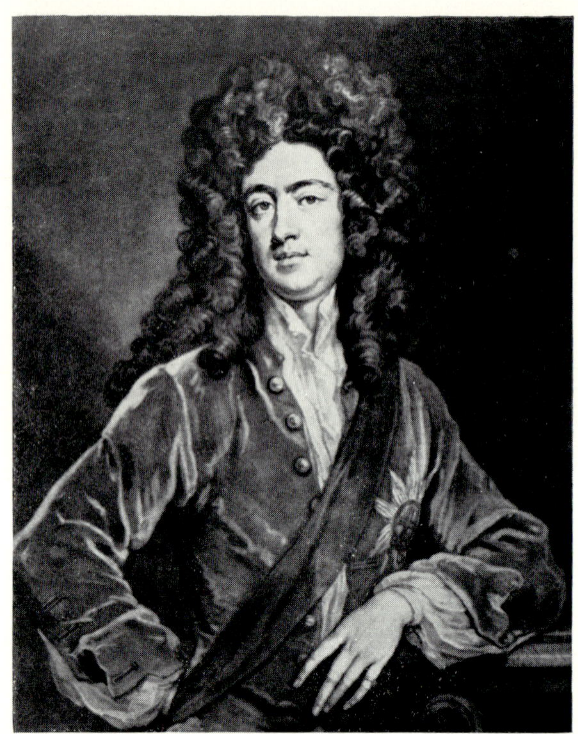

CHARLES LENNOX, SECOND DUKE OF RICHMOND, LENNOX AND AUBIGNY
The portrait by Kneller engraved by Faber
(*Reproduced by permission of the Syndics of the Fitzwilliam Museum, Cambridge*)

AN ARTIST'S IDEA OF THE NEW HOSPITAL WHEN COMPLETED
The painting by William Bellers in 1752 engraved by Chatelain and Toms
(*Reproduced by courtesy of the Trustees of the British Museum*)

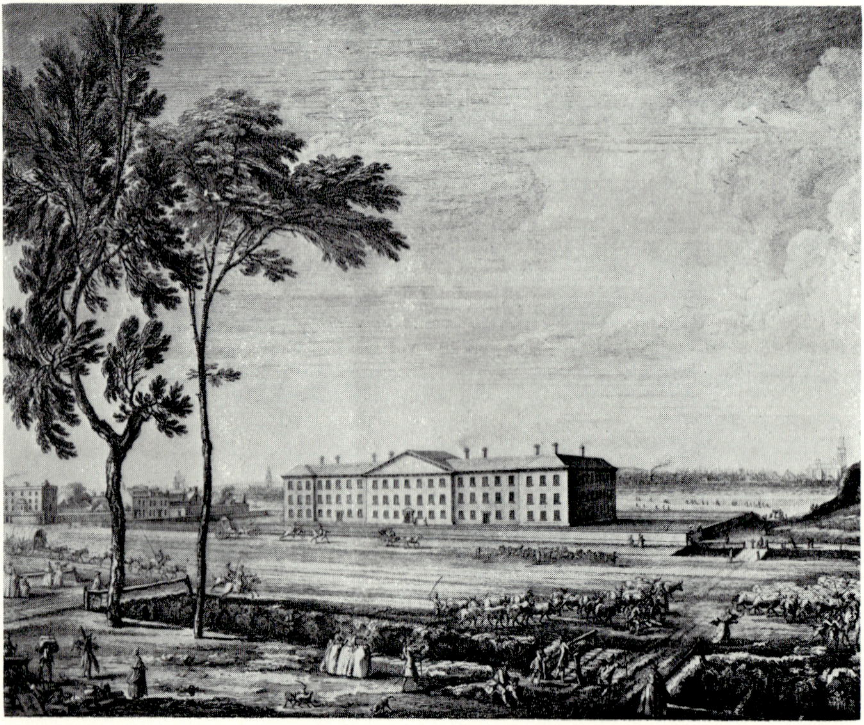

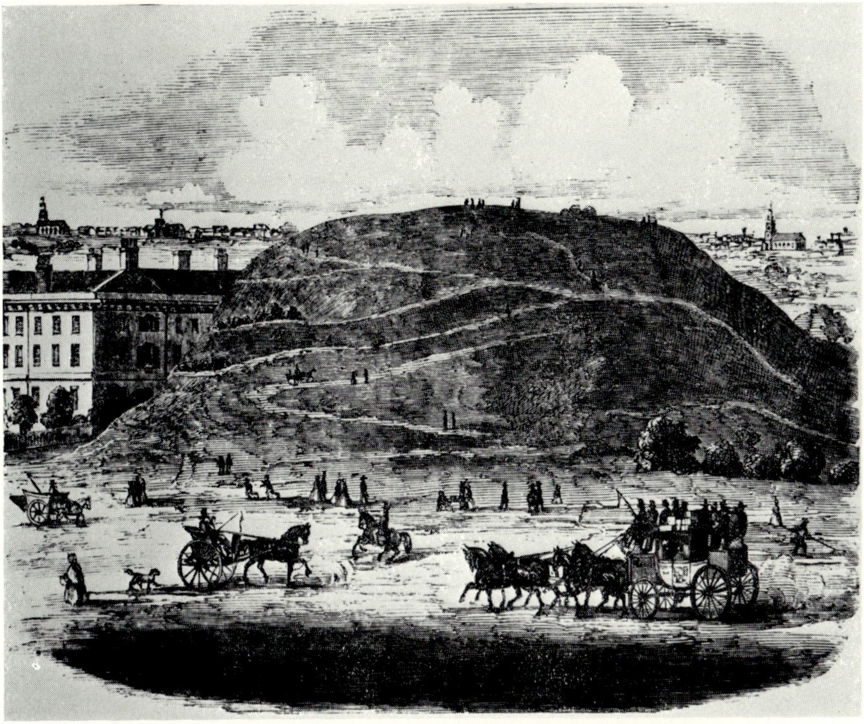

WHITECHAPEL MOUNT
SHOWING PART OF THE
HOSPITAL BEHIND IT
(*Reproduced by permission of
the Syndics of the Cambridge
University Press*)

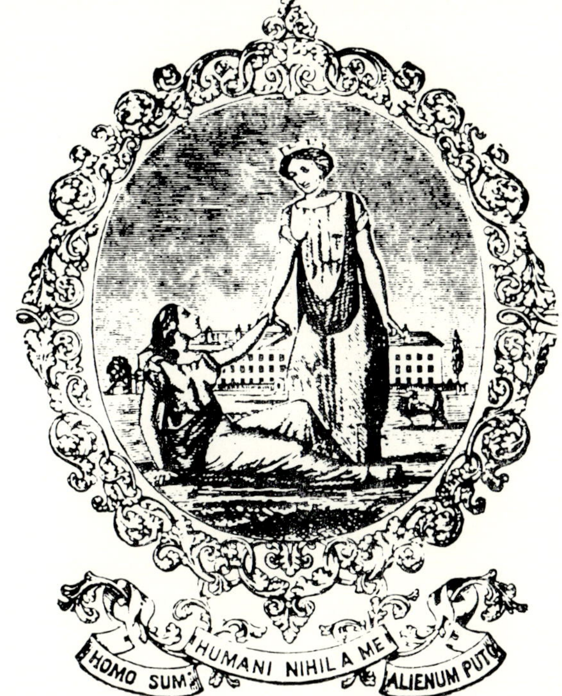

THE SEAL DESIGNED FOR
THE HOSPITAL BY JOHN
ELLICOTT AND ADAPTED
LATER AS THE CREST OF
THE MEDICAL COLLEGE

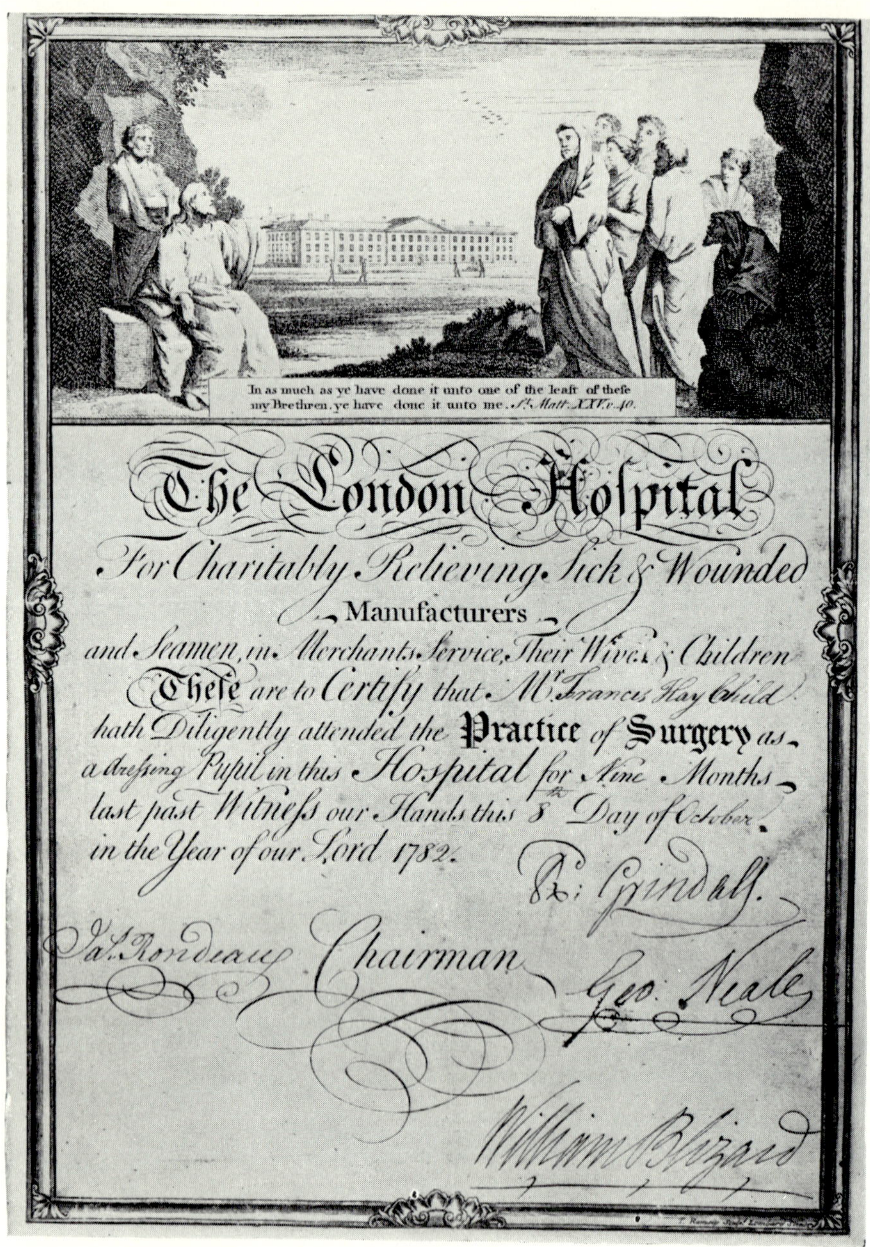

A PUPIL'S CERTIFICATE
The drawing at the top is by William Hogarth

but even then he always left directions with the apothecary or beadle as to how to get hold of him. If he could not be found, the beadle was under instructions to go in search of one of the surgeons extraordinary (i.e. extra-ordinary) as the assistant surgeons were still called. If no surgeon could be found, one of Mr Harrison's pupils would cope with the situation, an instance of which was quoted by the committee in their report. 'William Burridge was brought in about 3 in the afternoon for a Compound Fracture when your Surgeon in Ordinary was gone out of Town to Visit a patient. Whereupon Mr Wood (who had served Seven years with a Surgeon, and almost a year in the Hospital as a Pupil) first went to Mr Jones, your Surgeon Extraordinary, who was not in the Way, and then to a Surgeon Governor of this Hospital who was gone out of Town. Then Mr Wood, being unwilling to lose any more time, thought it better to Undertake this Patient himself with the assistance of the Other Pupils, as he apprehended himself Capable of it, and accordingly Set his Leg and did everything that Night. That Mr Harrison saw the Patient next day and found no occasion to make any alteration in what Mr Wood had done.'

All went well with William Burridge for about ten days. Then he started to shiver, 'and upon opening some abscesses which were found gathering in his leg, the Discharge was so great that he lost his appetite and Sunk under it, to which the then remarkable Warmth of the Weather was supposed to Contribute not a little. The setting the Leg the Night the patient came in was confirmed by the Nurse; It appearing he was very well used and that Mr Harrison ordered him Chicken, Fish, or anything else he could eat, and Large Nosegays to prevent his being affected by the Stench of his Leg. And that the Man was thankfull and Particularly so the day of his Death'.

Suggestions had also been made by some malign person that John Harrison was wont to use drugs in his private practice which really belonged to the hospital. The committee went into this. He did use them, they found, but the apothecary kept an accurate account of their cost which Harrison settled from time to time. He, the apothecary, admitted however that 'he had not kept any

Account of the Medicines delivered for Mr Harrison's Pupils, and Servants, [because] he had always thought it Customary to let them have what was Necessary for their own Illness, and Mr Harrison's Servants, as he was a governor, he considered as proper Objects of the Charity, and therefore he had attended and administered to them and that the Physicians also had had Medicines out of the Dispensary for their Servants'.

Laxity in respect of the rules of this kind was accepted without comment, but Mr Shields, the apothecary, came in for some criticism on other counts. He had left the fixing of 'Tickets on the Patients' Beds, Specifying their Names and Times of admission', for which he had been told he was responsible, to the nurses and watches and 'he did not keep a Book of the number of Patients on Each diet', nor the matrons informed as he had been instructed. He left all that to the steward. He confessed, too, that he had attended some of his friends but had been careful on all these occasions to see that his absence had not been prejudicial to the interests of the hospital in any way. On a few occasions he had, it is true, 'given Physick out of the Dispensary to some poor Relations and Others, whom he considered as proper Objects of Compassion, wherein he had in some Measure transgressed the Letter of the Law but that he had been induced to do it by the Ties of Relationship and Friendship'. For this he now 'humbly hoped to be excused', promising 'to avoid everything of like kind for the future'. When he went out, he had always left a note in the dispensary to say where he would be going and, 'except on very Extraordinary Occasions he had not lain out without leave for two years past; and that he had always taken care to appoint a proper Person to officiate for him'. He went round the wards, he said, three or four times a day, but not at nine in the morning as strictly required of him. This, he alleged, 'was Inconvenient, by Reason that the Wards were then cleaning and the Women dressing themselves'. These were minor matters. What did matter was his professional ability. 'As to Mr Shields's general Character as an Apothecary', wrote the committee of inquiry, 'we find from the concurrent Testimony of Your Physicians and Surgeon in Ordinary that he is a very able Apothecary, exceeded by None, and the Physicians declared that he is likewise a very good Chymist, always in the way, and ready to assist in all Cases.'

The rest of the staff came out of the inquiry well. 'As to the Reverend Mr Audley, we find that he constantly reads Prayers at the Hospital every Tuesday and Saturday; that he always visits and prays by Such of the Patients as desire it, and administers the Sacrament to Such of them, as upon inquiry into their Lives and Conversation, he thinks fitly Qualified to receive it.' They found the Bishop of Sodor & Man's *Christian Instructions* posted in every ward. They also inquired into the behaviour of the secretary, steward, matrons, nurses, watches, beadles and apothecary's man, and found them all 'agreeable to the Rules of the House relating to them Respectively'.

Even the students came out of the inquiry with flying colours. The dressing pupils had long become a cog in the wheels of the hospital machine. For some time already, under *Standing Orders*, one of them had been 'required to attend in the Hospital constantly day and night and diet with one of the Matrons'. Now, 'as the daily business of the house often detained the pupils until 4 or 5 o'clock in the afternoon and sometimes longer', another pupil had been ordered to dine in the house 'so that its Business might be done without delay'.

The walking pupils played no part in what was going on. They were mere spectators, more like post-graduate students in an undergraduate teaching hospital today. Some had already taken a theoretical degree in medicine at a university and were now gaining practical experience before being examined orally for the licentiateships of the College of Physicians which conferred on them the right to practise 'physick' within seven miles of the City. Others had been dressers at other hospitals, or apprentices to surgeons in practice, and were waiting to take the examination for membership of Surgeons' Hall before setting up in practice themselves or getting jobs on ships or in the army.

Pupils paid their fees to the member of the staff under whom they worked as dressers or who had got them permission to walk the wards, but all were required to conform to the rules and regulations of the hospital and enjoined by the house committee 'to be tender to the patients'. This system had soon caused trouble. The dressers in particular came to see themselves as servants, not of the hospital, but of the surgeons who had taken them on and to whom they were paying their fees, so the committee had been forced into action. 'Whereas several Inconveniences have arisen by Pupils Misbehaving and neglect of Duty, greatly owing to their thinking themselves subject only to the orders of the particular Surgeon with whom they are entered, Agreed that all the Pupils shall be under the Direction of all or either of the Surgeons, and in future all advantages arising from the taking of Pupils shall be distributed equally between the Surgeons.'

There was still an absolute dividing line between medicine and surgery. Pupils never came to study both. Nor was there an opportunity for them to learn anatomy – for that they had to go to one of the private medical schools or to Surgeons' Hall. Nor were any lectures allowed in the hospital. John Harrison had been given permission to read lectures in the court room in 1747 but when Henry Thompson (as assistant surgeon) now applied for similar permission, he was told that the hospital had been founded and was being maintained for treating 'poor objects' and that he must 'find another Place for the Purpose'. The governors also rationed the staff in respect of pupils, the number of dressers to be kept down to the minimum necessary to do the work of the hospital.

The pupils were a rough lot but, as in the case of the nurses, it is the offenders who figure in the minutes. Sometimes there were mitigating circumstances. Prescott Street must have been hot and stuffy in July. 'Complaints having been made against the Pupils for going into the cold Bath and misbehaving there, Ordered that in future no Pupil have Liberty to go into the cold Bath on any Pretence whatever.' A more serious matter was reported later. 'Complaint having been made against Mr Edward Towsey, the Surgeon's Pupil for the Week, the Committee, on examining William Ross, a patient in Devonshire's Ward [so called after the Duke who had succeeded the Duke of Richmond as president on the death of the latter] found that the said Edwd. Towsey came home last Monday between Twelve and One o'clock (at night) and greatly abused the Watch, took away her Lamp, and opened the Surgery Window, and let in Mr Kam another pupil, and two Strange Women who continued in the House a Considerable time making a great Noise and disturbance.' Then they examined Betty Muckelroy, the watch who let them in, who declared 'that on her saying she had no Candle for him, he cursed and Swore at her greatly, and threatened to Kick her about the passage. And Ann Brown, the Watch for Johns ward, confirmed his bad behaviour and about an hour after thinking she smell Fire, got a Patient to go down with her to see if Mr Towseys light was out, and saw something standing in a Shirt which much frightened her. The said Towsey told her next morning that it was Mr Kam she had seen in his shirt, and that he had a Shovel in his hand to knock down any One who should attempt to come into his Room.' On being accused Mr Towsey acknowledged 'the whole of the Above, except the Women being in the House, which he denied, alleging they were only at the Window'. The 'said Towsey' was discharged from all further attendance at the hospital.

In 1753 Henry Dobson died, creating a vacancy for a surgeon extraordinary. The same machinery was adopted to replace him as on previous occasions. There were seven candidates. Four hundred and sixty-one governors voted and Richard Grindall was elected by a majority of 206 over his nearest rival. Shortly after this, on account of John Harrison's rapidly failing health, the governors advertised for yet another assistant surgeon. Three gentlemen applied this time and at the election, the Marquis of Granby in the chair, the same large number of governors balloted and fifty-three noblemen and ladies sent proxies. Gabriel Risolière, a Huguenot refugee living in Spitalfields, who had learnt his craft as an apprentice in London, was elected by a large majority.

Shortly after this, John Harrison, virtual founder of the hospital, died at the age of thirty-five at his house in Savage Gardens, Tower Hill. 'For the Encrease and Support of that Charity,' wrote the *Public Advertiser*, a leading newspaper of that day, 'he had spent almost his whole time and been at very great expense ever since its first institution which he was principally concerned in'. He had continued working up to the end, but the last years of his life had been clouded by the petty jealousy of certain colleagues. Further, as the number of governors increased, and the medical staff became larger, he had been less and less influential in the affairs of the charity.

'To my friend the Reverend Matthew Audley,' he had written in his will, 'I give and bequeath my best diamond Ring, one Taper Silver Candle stick, six Silver Table Spoons and ten Guinease in Money as a small acknowledgement of the Affection and Friendship he has always shown me; unto my late apprentice, Mr Henry Thompson, my two small silver Candle Sticks, Snuffers and Stand marked with a Cock, and one Taper candle Stick with all my Books, Instruments and Preparations for Surgery.' To the secretary, steward, two matrons and beadle he left one guinea each. Then, after other small legacies, he left the whole residue of his estate to 'his dearest friend, Mr Shute Adams, of Fleet St., London, druggust'. To the hospital he left nothing. 'As I have spent', he wrote, 'a considerable part of my fortune, life, ease and health in the service of it, I can only leave my good wishes for the prosperity of that Charity, whose interests I have always pursued at the expense of my own.'

Henry Thompson, now a member of the surgical staff, had difficulty in getting his instruments. Did they not really belong to the charity as an institution rather than to John Harrison personally? Some said the latter, but Thompson succeeded in proving his title to them, although not all the committee, it seems, were ever quite convinced. Anyhow there was to be no doubt as to the ownership of the surgical instruments in future. 'Agreed that there be an Inventory taken of all the Chirurgical Instruments belonging to the Charity, and that a proper Box or Locker be made to keep them in and a good Lock with two Keys be provided for the said Box, one key to be held by Mrs Broad, Matron, and the other by the surgery man who also is to take particular Care of the said Instruments and, if at any time any part of them should be missing, he inform the Committee at the next Meeting.'

Mr Shields, the apothecary, had got off lightly at the hands of the committee and had been allowed an apprentice, who was 'at liberty to follow the Box' (i.e. the box containing instruments carried before a surgeon as he went round his wards), and was to attend all surgical operations, but was 'debarred the liberty of bleeding or dressing any Patient whatsoever'. This saved Mr Shields a certain amount of work, but was a concession which may have been a mistake. When a committee was appointed to inquire into the working of the dispensary, they found it in chaos. The 'elaboratory man' had 'hired himself to go Surgeon of a ship to Greenland' and the drugs, it seems, were not being looked after properly. Nor were 'the medicines being properly prepared'. His statements, too, were found to be inaccurate, even untruthful. The 'physical committee' had not been called for over a year. On many occasions, too, he could not be found, 'often lying abroad without Leave'. So, having been found out, Mr Shields saved the committee further trouble by tendering his resignation.

A new apothecary now had to be found, so 'the physical committee' met and examined a large number of applicants 'in their knowledge of Drugs, their Composition and Use', the actual election attracting as much interest as one to the senior medical staff. Over three hundred governors voted, peers and ladies again sending proxies, and Mr James Baittaile was elected on the same terms as Mr Shields.

The patients were kept under strict discipline. They were not allowed to leave the house 'on any account whatever' although, under exceptional circumstances, they could get a permit from the apothecary. They were not allowed 'to play at Cards, Dice, or any other Games, or smoake in the wards or anywhere else in the House'; to 'sit up after nine at farthest in the Winter and ten in Summer'; to 'send for or receive Provisions of any sort, Spiritous or other Liquors'; to 'swear, curse or use abusive Language or behave themselves indecently'; all 'under pain of Expulsion' and any patient discharged was never to be re-admitted. They were required to 'take such Medicines as are ordered by the Physicians' and 'Submit to the Operation judged necessary'. When sufficiently well they were expected 'to attend divine service on Sunday'; to 'assist the Nurses and Watches in taking care of the others, in cleaning the Wards, Washing, ironing and mending Linen for the use of the House or in such other manner that the Matrons shall think fit'.

These rules, like all rules, were sometimes broken. A patient would go out, come back drunk and 'cause a Disturbance in the Wards'. One was discharged for 'indecent Behaviour'. Elizabeth Storey, recommended by Mr Martin, 'ridiculed the Physicians and Surgeons and took a Vomit of her own accord [a strange thing to do, it would seem] which was designed for another patient' and was discharged. Mr Martin was informed accordingly. Another maintained that 'his Sheets were foul and his Bed lousy', but on inquiry his complaint was found to be 'frivolous', and, as 'his behaviour had been very Irregular the whole time he was in the House', the committee got rid of him as quickly as they could. Extenuating circumstances were always taken into account. On one occasion, for instance, a patient in the lock 'layed out all Night contrary to the Regulations but, as he confessed his Error and it appearing that he had lately lost a leg in the Defence of his Country, Agreed to continue him on his asking Pardon'.

Before any patient was discharged for refusing treatment every precaution was taken to ensure that he had the benefit of the best medical advice. The committee laid down that 'in any case of difficulty or danger' all the surgeons were to consult together and the majority decision carried out. So when George Delaney, a boy with a white swelling of his knee and caries of his tibia, was admitted under Mr Grindall, he 'summoned a consultation of several Surgeons of character who were unanimous in their Opinion of taking off the Limb'. His parents refused consent and, when this was reported to the committee, it was 'Moved the said George Delaney be immediately discharged'. Further, no 'capital operation', they said, was ever to be performed 'except by the orders and with the consent of the majority of the Physicians and Surgeons of the hospital', another advance, it would seem, in the physician–surgeon relationship. Due notice of an operation, too, was always 'to be given to the other surgeons for their attendance, save under circumstances of absolute necessity'.

When a patient died his body was carried into the lobby, and then over to the dead-house, while the steward notified the next of kin, in the hope that they would come and take it away, as each burial cost the charity 13s. When no reply was received, the clothing and personal effects of the deceased were sold 'to the best Bidder in the Presence of the Governors', and the proceeds put in the poor box, a practice which led to the impression that the infirmary always kept the effects of the deceased and landed the governor with the expense of burying many bodies which relatives, had they not thought that, would have buried themselves. The committee was therefore forced into publishing a notice to the effect that, if relatives wished to bury the deceased, they would always have their clothes and personal effects returned.

Bodies were sometimes smuggled out of the hospital, the committee soon discovered, to be sold for dissection to one of the private schools of anatomy which were now springing up. Even the surgeons were not innocent in this matter. 'The committee being informed that dead Bodys have been carried out of this Hospital contrary to the Rules of the Charity, they proceeded to inquire into the Truth of the said Information, and having Examined John Cushee and John Smith, the Two Beadles, They acknowledged that on Friday night they did carry out the body of a Woman in a Hamper by order of Mr Grindall, and by him desired to leave it at the House of Mr Douglas, a Surgeon in Cannon Street. That being stop'd by Two Custom house Officers on Tower Hill they were carried before Col. Willoughby (who being Satisfied by Oath made before Him that the Woman died a natural Death in this Hospital), they were discharged, and brought the Body back again, which was next day Burried in White Chapel Burrying Ground at the expense of this Charity. They confessed that they had carried or sent out to the Surgeons within Nine Months past Four Bodys.'

This had to be stopped. The surgeons were hauled up before the committee and 'did acknowledge that they had had some Bodys carried out of the Hospital to their own Houses, or to Mr Douglas's, but that they did not know it was against the Laws of the Charity. Whereupon they promised Strict Conformity to the Same.' The beadles made no attempt to plead ignorance. They were 'reprimanded' from the chair and promised 'Strict Obedience to the Laws for the future, and that they would never Offend in the like manner again'.

Trouble, and expense too, was sometimes caused by the coroner refusing to give permission for a body to be buried until 'he had sat on it'. His fee for this was 13s. On one occasion, a Swiss soldier died in the infirmary but could not be buried because the coroner would not give the necessary permission 'until he had sat on it' and the parish would not pay his fee. So, 'the Corps becoming obnoxious', the secretary was instructed to write to him as follows:

> *The Governors of this Charity have ordered me to acquaint you that they were in Hope that you would have granted an order for the Burial of a Swiss soldier (who is become a prodigious Nuisance) without putting them to any Expense, as they have nothing but the Benefactions of charitable people, but they still hope you will be so good as to send it by the Bearer, who has orders to satisfy you if you are not inclined to save the Charity that Expense.*

The coroner continued adamant and the bearer paid him his fee.

The cost of getting patients home was defrayed by the hospital if necessary. Grace Harley got a shilling to enable her to get to Stratford in Essex; John Kelly, 'in a consumption', the cost of a coach to Shadwell; Isaac Goulding, 'recommended by Mrs Lucy Alie, and this day discharged relieved of a dropsy', 2s. 6d. for one to Soho. One got his coach paid to Petticoat Lane; another his expenses to Barnet, 'he, being very poor and friendless'. Sometimes they had to be sent home even farther afield. 'Ordered that James Bull, an accidental Patient, discharged this day cured of an Abscess in his leg, have money to pay his necessary Expenses to Chesterford in Cambridgeshire, and that the Steward do agree with the Waggoner for the same.' Nor would the committee send patients home entirely destitute. John Edwin, Esq., a governor, left a will 'wherein he Bequeathed £20 p.ann. for 10 years to be distributed among the poorest of the Patients when they are discharged who, although Cured of their Diseases, being sent out of a comfortable Place and having no immediate Employment or perhaps not well enough to work at it, are destitute of food, firing and lodging, not to exceed 10s. to any one patient'.

No patient was allowed to remain in the infirmary for more than two months without the permission of the house committee and the demand for the beds was now so great that we find the committee pressing the physicians to get their patients home. In their eyes, the physicians were often not strict enough and, before long, they appointed three of their own number to go round the wards from time to time and decide for themselves which of those patients who had been in the hospital for a very long time could be sent out, yet another example of the degree to which the lay governors of this date controlled and disciplined the professional staff.

Looking back now on these years, too, we are surely driven to admire, not only the quantity and quality of the work which the lay committee put into the administration of the infirmary, but also, although they had to be strict, the compassion which genuinely inspired it.

4

Coming of Age

In his sermon at the festival the Bishop of Worcester had emphasized the decrepit condition and costly upkeep of the houses in Prescott Street. Now he had followed up his words by action, and the governors could write round 'to the nobility' to inform them that 'the Lord Bishop, out of his great regard for the Infirmary, has opened a Subscription for raising a Fund to erect a new Building by the time the Lease of the present Premises shall Expire: which will then be too old and Ruinous to continue in longer'. The bishop himself, they were told, had sent the charity 'a draft on his Goldsmith for £20'. They now solicited their generous support. There was also to be a charity concert. 'Agreed that Mr Handel be desired to favour the Governors with a Performance for the Benefit of the Hospital to be applied to the Building Account at the great Room at the Swan in Cornhill, the said Room and the usual Accommodation thereof, being offered *gratis* by Mr Comyns.'

This fund stood at over £5000, but the appeal which had raised it had already lost its initial momentum and subscriptions were now coming in only slowly. It was time, the committee thought, to urge the governors into further efforts. 'As the expenses attending the Tenements at present occupied leave no Room to doubt', they wrote in their quarterly report, 'they will be incapable of further Use at or before the Expiration of the present Lease, your Committee apprehend we cannot too early secure a proper Piece of Ground for Building.' There was more than enough money for that already, vested in the hands of the Trustees. There were 'convenient places for that Purpose', they said, 'to be had which may not Offer should there be any Delay'. Until the governors had found a site, too, how could they ask the surveyor to draw plans for a new hospital? Until they had got those, how could they commission an artist to produce a drawing of what it would look like when finished? This, they said, should be 'engraved on a copper Plate and copies thereof dispersed among the Governors and others inclinable to promote it'. Only in this way would the appeal be galvanized back into life and sub-scriptions start coming in again. The governors should appoint a special committee, they said, 'to Examine into and procure such a Piece of Land in the Cheapest and best Manner'. They con-cluded with a word of caution. Prices were bound to rise when it was known what the hospital was up to. This committee would need to proceed with 'great Management, Secrecy and Expedi-tion'.

The court were quick to see the wisdom of this advice and appointed a special committee, under the chairmanship of the Earl of Macclesfield, President of the Royal Society, mathemati-cian and astronomer, and member of Parliament since 1742, to find a site. They got down to work at once, briefing Mr Main-waring, the hospital surveyor, as to what they had in mind and asking him to start looking round for a suitable site without delay.

In spite of the optimism of the house committee, months passed before he had anything to report. 'The only Piece of Ground', he now told them, 'apprehended suitable for this occasion is situate near the River and commonly known as White Chapel Mount and the Mount Field.' This lay about a mile from Aldgate just south of the main highway leading from Essex into the City. To the north stood a row of houses and, to the north of them, was the Ducking Pond and Ducking Pond Lane; farther north was the hamlet of Bethnal Green, still out in open country. To the south agricultural land stretched down to the river and the docks. To the east lay Mile End Old Town; to the west the White Chapel. The Mount was a natural mound which had been fortified by Parliament against the King in the Civil

War, and on the top of which had been piled much of the debris from the great fire of 1666. It now stood, it was said, over 300 feet high and from the top of it an extensive view could be obtained.

The Mount and the Mount Field just to the east of it, Mr Mainwaring explained, were held on lease from the City by Mr Worrall (described in the minutes as a 'Bilder') for sixty years, of which fifty-three were still to run, at an annual rent of £26. The City in turn held it, and more land besides, on lease from Lady Wentworth for a term of five hundred years of which only sixty years had run. Mr Worrall had said in conversation that he would part with his lease for £750. Mr Mainwaring 'apprehended that he would take £600'. So the committee, 'deeming it [the site] of sufficient Size', appointed three of their number to negotiate with Mr Worrall and, although he now said he would part with his lease for £500, the committee thought even this too much. They sheered off and instructed Mr Mainwaring to go on looking round to see what else he could find.

Many possible sites were inspected by the committee but again and again something ruled one after the other out. A piece of ground in East Smithfield was rejected because it was 'too small' and 'the Situation not so Suitable'. Perhaps it was thought too near St Bartholomew's. An attractive site on Tower Hill 'commonly known as Ditch Side could not be Purchased at present'. An 'entire Field' near 'the Watch House' on the Bethnal Green side of the Hackney Road was 'apprehended too far from Town for the Physicians and Surgeons to attend'. A house in Aldersgate was considered 'confined too much in point of Air'. Among other sites, one in Whitechapel was rejected as 'being too near the White Lead Works which might be injurious to the Health of the Patients'.

After eighteen months of hard work, in fact, the committee came to the conclusion that the only thing to do was to come to terms with Mr Worrall, although of course he would now have put up his price, and they eventually had to agree to give him £800 for his lease, provided that the City were prepared to lease the land to them at the end of it. So the next step was to 'petition' the Lord Mayor 'praying' that the rest of the City's lease from Lady Wentworth might be assigned to the infirmary. The request was received favourably. What is more, as the Committee of City Lands advised against parting with the Mount itself on long lease, the City agreed to reduce the ground rent for the field to £15, an arrangement which suited the governors. The Mount could have been little use to them. These details settled, as the hospital was not yet a corporate body in law, they nominated six of their number to hold the field in trust on behalf of the charity. Further, an unexpected opportunity now arose to buy up land to the immediate south. 'Mr Knight's moiety of the Freehold of the Red Lyon Farm and the Copyhold adjoining', part of the estate of the late Bailey Heath, Esq., and comprising ten acres of agricultural land, suddenly came on the market. After interminable legal complications the governors succeeded in acquiring it for £1442.

The special committee appointed to find a site now handed over to a building committee under the chairmanship of Sir Peter Warren, who had been second in command to Anson of the Battle of Cape Finisterre and was now reputed the richest commoner in England. This, too, got down to work at once; 'Agreed to desire Mr Mainwaring to prepare plans for a Building fit for the reception of two hundred Patients with proper Offices and with a Reserve to increase that Building as circumstances may require it'.

Meanwhile, the house committee had to face the problem of the prevention of theft from the property they had now acquired. 'Fences round White Chapel Mount have been frequently Broken down and the Pales carried away', they reported to the governors. Some of these thieves were caught. John Chambers, who 'caught the Thief that stole the Pales from White Chapel Mount and attended 4 days at Hicks Hall during the Prosecution', got 19s. as a reward. What punishment was meted out to the thief is not recorded. Before long they were forced to employ night watchmen, and a year later we find Mr Mainwaring informing them that 'one of the Men whom he employed to watch the Fences at White Chapel Mount had caught one Thomas Wilkinson with three of the Pales he had stolen from the same Fence'. So Fotherley Baker was 'desired to Prosecute the said Thomas Wilkinson at Quarter Sessions at Hicks Hall tomorrow'.

Mr Mainwaring submitted four alternative plans for a new hospital out of which the building committee chose his numbers two and three to lay before the governors. The former envisaged three detached blocks linked by colonnades; the latter a central block, running east and west parallel with the main road, with two wings extending out to the south. Both would provide for nearly four hundred beds. So the court met at Prescott Street on 25 September 1757 and came down unanimously in favour of plan number two; that is to say, three detached blocks.

Mr Mainwaring now started to examine the ground. 'As far as he had gone, it appeared to be all dug out of Gravell and filled up again with Hog and Rubbish, except some part next the Road which he found to be natural Ground, and he apprehended he shall soon find a proper Bed for the Foundation fit for a Building.' Meanwhile the committee became beset by second thoughts about the plan the governors had chosen. It was certainly the most ostentatious. The committee would have preferred Mr Mainwaring's number three, and now 'thought it their Duty to the Charity maturely to Examine and Reconsider the Plan laid before the General Court at their last Meeting, to the Intent that that if any Alteration would appear to be either necessary or advisable, we might in time apply to the Court for their Opinion and Directions'.

So many alterations in this plan did in fact appear to the committee to be both 'necessary and advisable' that they asked the long-suffering Mr Mainwaring to draw up another and this, a modification of his original number three, was submitted to the governors. 'All the wards would have a southern aspect,' said the committee in presenting it, 'which, in the Opinion of the Physicians and Surgeons, was most desirable for the Patients.' They would be shielded, too, from 'the dust and cold winds' of the road. 'By the continuity of the said Building,' they continued, 'your Physicians, Surgeons and Apothecary could at all times and in all Seasons attend your Patients in all parts of it without the

Danger and Inconvenience to which they might be exposed by their Attendance at different detached parts as proposed by the former Plan.' One continuous building, they argued, would be 'in its nature stronger and more lasting than the same quantity divided into three separate Blocks', and 'also avoid the expense of colonnades'. They recommended setting the hospital back from the road with an area of 70 feet between for the Governors' coaches and chariots which 'cannot but, in our Opinion, have a very good Effect', and 'permit the planting of Trees'. The governors were convinced by these arguments and discarded the idea of blocks linked by colonnades, which they had adopted only three months before. They now accepted *nem con* the more practical single-block design recommended by their committee.

The idea of a new hospital had captured the imagination of the governors. Money began to roll in and a determined effort was now made to make the festival of 1752 an overwhelming success. Scaffolding was put up in the church for 'a Band of Musick' and three thousand copies of the anthem printed. The *Gentleman's Magazine* waxed enthusiastic. 'At a sermon preached at *Christ-Church Newgate Street* on account of the London Hospital was a most numerous appearance of Ladies; the collection was very large there, and at Merchant Tailor's Hall the Marquis of Hartington paid in a benefaction of £300 from Matthew Lamb, Esq. as did John Gore, Esq., £150 from two persons unknown; the whole amount £2,093.' This, a record, was attributed largely to 'the Musickal Performance' of which the Lord Bishop was 'graciously pleased to express his complete approval'.

At midsummer the building committee 'had the Pleasure to inform the Court that the first Planck was laid and the Foundations of the Hospital begun on the 11th day of June instant'. This event was also reported in the *Gentleman's Magazine*. 'The first stone was laid of the foundation of the new *London hospital* near *White-Chapel Mount* in the presence of the Duke of Bedford, Sir Peter Warren and divers other persons of distinction.' Building progressed only slowly, for the committee was compelled to proceed in stages as money became available. Mr Mainwaring had estimated that laying the foundations and carrying 'the shell'

C

of the front block up to first-floor level would cost £5000, and the financial position did not allow the committee to think in terms of going further than that for the moment; when autumn came, all building operations had to be suspended and steps taken to protect what had been built already. 'Ordered two new Sewers to be made directly to carry away the Water that may fall into the Building and which will carry away the Sullidge water from the building when finished.' The whole structure, too, had to be covered over temporarily to protect it from frost. This proved an expensive item and throughout the winter watchmen had to be employed to prevent damage and theft.

In the spring, building started again and it was now 'the unanimous Wish of the Committee that after the usual Sermon at the next Annual Festival [6 April 1753], the President, Governors and other Gentlemen be desired to go in procession to view the new Buildings and from thence to the Hall for dinner'. So 'Mr Mainwaring was desired to order the Ground to be cleared for the Coaches to pass' and, when the day came, a cavalcade headed by the new president, the Duke of Devonshire, proceeded from St Mary's Church, Whitechapel, to Whitechapel Mount. Thence, all having had a good look, it returned to Merchant Taylors' Hall where over four hundred sat down to dinner. Gift tickets had been distributed to ladies and the company included Lady Warren – Sir Peter had recently died – Mrs Parsons, owner of the public house in Prescott Street, and Mrs Alie who had given £500 to the building fund 'to be deemed the intended Benefaction of her late Brother, Richard Leman Esq., deceased', the first landlord of the infirmary in Prescott Street. The collection in the church and at the hall amounted to £1536.

Mr Mainwaring now estimated that the centre block could be carried up another storey and roofed over for £5300, and the committee risked ordering him to proceed. So in spite of a wet autumn the shell of the building was finished by the end of the year, but they now found themselves 'under the greatest Difficulty to pay the Workmen'. The good name of the charity was bound to suffer if they defaulted, and there was much anxiety on this account. Then the situation was saved, as they reported to the governors, 'by our Vice-President and Treasurer who advanced without Interest £350 each and Payed the same into the hands of your Bankers for the use of your Committee'.

When the building season came round again in the spring, after repaying these loans, there was only £276 left in the building account, but in spite of this the committee risked entering into contracts for flooring the centre block, the situation being eased for the moment by Mr Gregory and other governors offering 'to lay one of the Floors entirely at their own Expense'. To all intents and purposes, however, progress with the new building in Whitechapel had come to a complete standstill.

In the meanwhile the tenements in Prescott Street had sunk into a deplorable state: 'Ordered that the Ceiling under the Steward's room be lathed and plastered to prevent the Sand coming through.' Worse was soon happening in Mrs Broad's kitchen, the sand coming through from the wards above. Rain-water also started to flood into Mrs Gouy's. The apothecary complained 'that the Water from the cold Bath overflowed into the Elaboratory so that the Man cannot do his Work'. Then Mr Lacey Roberts, who lived next door, objected to the 'soil' from the 'Necessary House' oozing through into his garden 'causing such a stench that they could not bear it, his Landlord threatening to prosecute the Charity if not directly Remedied'. The owners of the houses in Chamber Street at the back of the infirmary also threatened legal action against the hospital because the cesspool was still overflowing into it. Mr Mainwaring was consulted again, but the only solution of this problem which he now had to offer (his previous solution having failed) was to dig a drain to the common sewer in the main road. This would cost £260, money which could be much better spent, the committee thought, on the new building.

The crisis in the affairs of the charity, long foreseen, had in fact been reached. The governors were now in a desperate dilemma. The old infirmary in Prescott Street stank to high heaven and its floors were in danger of collapse. All work on the new hospital had stopped. They were without money to repair and maintain the former and at the same time go ahead with the latter, so an extraordinary meeting of the court was called for 27 November 1754 to review the whole situation.

At this meeting the committee submitted estimates for the completion of the centre block. The cellar, they said, with its stairway, long passage, two laundries and waiting-room would cost £1006 1s. 11d. Finishing the ground floor so as to provide an entrance hall, bleeding-room, surgery, cold bath, apothecary's shop, physicians' room and two wards with lobbies, privies and sculleries, fitted with sinks, would cost £1519 10s. 8d. The first floor, with stairs up to it, providing two wards similarly equipped, the court room and rooms for the matron, surgeons, surgeon's man and steward, would cost another £1562 3s. 9d. Finishing off part of the second floor to provide two wards would cost £381 17s. 6d. This added up to £4529 3s. 10d. 'which Sum', the committee said, 'will so far complete the Centre as to enable you to remove the patients into the new Building and will add to your present Number of 132 beds (at Prescott Street) 29 which will make 161 beds'. Another £539 would be required to complete the third storey. This would provide another 51 beds, bringing the total complement of beds up to 212.

These estimates left the attics unfinished. They would cost £285 'exclusive of the Theatre'. Nor did they include 'the two Doric Frontispieces with Colloms of Portland Stone with curved Trusses', that Mr Mainwaring had designed, or 'the Brickwall and Sewer in the Front, and the Walls, to inclose the grounds, with Portland Stone coping to the wall next the Road and Balls to the Piers of the Iron Gates'. All that was aesthetic luxury. 'However necessary it may be, yet in amounting to so large a Sum as £2562, your Committee think it incumbent on them to inform the General Court thereof, but apprehend it more for the Interest of this Charity to Compleat the most Useful parts first.'

The situation was desperate. The new hospital must be finished so that Prescott Street, which continued a drain on the financial resources of the charity – it had cost over £2000 to maintain during the past year – could be relinquished. Nearly £2000 was put down round the table and the governors unanimously agreed to start a new 'Subscription' – we would call it an appeal – and, as it was thought that 'it would be agreeable to many Gentlemen to be waited on in order to receive their Donations to the Building', twenty-six of their number were appointed a 'Deputation'. This was organized on a regional basis. Each member of it undertook to wait on all likely subscribers in his own district.

In the spring of 1756, after an unhappy interlude of over a year, building started again. The attics were now to be finished and the gaunt 'shell' roofed over and fitted up within. Work continued uninterrupted throughout the year. Soon after Christmas the windows were being glazed and in the following spring the committee began thinking in terms of furnishing the rooms according to their allocation under Mainwaring's plan.

There were to be two wards on each of the three floors, and after their experience at Prescott Street the committee would have liked to have furnished them with iron bedsteads. This proved too expensive. They were compelled to revert to wood but decided to make a clean sweep of all the old bedding and buy new. The nurse on each ward was to sleep in a room just outside it. This was provided with 'an iron bedstead, a feather bed and bolster, sheets and pillows, two blankets and coverlet, two rush-bottom chairs, a deal table, a two-leaf cloathes horse and an iron door lock and key'. The committee also ordered 'closets', i.e. sitting-rooms, to be made in each of the wards 'for the con-venience of the Nurses'. The night nurses were to sleep in the attics. 'Ordered that a Room in the Roof of the New House be prepared for the use of the Watches.' This was provided with 'four four post bedsteads, feather beds and bolsters, blankets, sheets and coverlets, a range and spare bar, a wood bottom chair and an iron rimmed door lock and key'.

The operating theatre, as planned, now looked likely to prove unsatisfactory. 'It having been reported that the center room in the Attick Storey designed for a Theatre will not serve for that Purpose Your committee desired Mr Mainwaring to order a sky-light to be fixed in the roof of the House for a room with two pairs of Stairs for the use of the Surgeons as a Theatre.' This was provided with 'an iron range and fender, an amputation table, mattress and pillow, an instrument table and operating table, an arm chair and stool, a large deal press with doors, lock and keys, an iron rimmed lock with brass knobs and key and . . .' – here a page has been torn out of the only inventory of its equipment at this date surviving.

The bleeding-room was fitted up with 'a Pump, a Sink, two elbow Chairs and a Ladle with a chain for the Patients to drink out of'; the surgery with 'a large winscot Table, Blinds for the Windows, six chairs and a large Stone for mixing ointments on'. The equipment of the apothecary's shop was elaborate, among the many items listed: 'a cast iron Bath, stove with fender, shovel, tongs and poker, a wanscot pillar and drawtable, a wanscot desk and drawers, a lead pump with iron work compleat, a sink and stand, a large bell mettle mortar, iron pestel and wood stand, a chair and stool, a closet with folding doors, lock and key, a pair of copper scales, and sundry brass weights, wanscot dining table, two pewter basons and all the necessary drawers, pigeon holes and jars'. The physicians' room was furnished *de luxe*. The committee ordered 'a pantheon stove, a steel fender and fire irons, mahogany frame folding window blinds, six Yew tree arm chairs, a mahogany three drawer library table with a green cloath, a plaster ink stand desk, a hand bell, an eight-day clock in a walnut tree case, a mahogany dining table, two deal cupboards, two door springs and two iron bound door locks and keys'. The court room on the first floor was furnished with a 'register stove, a wanscot bookcase, a wrought iron chest, a shoe cupboard, twenty mahogany chairs with leather seats, an elbow chair with footboard, a committee table on casters, a hand bell and mallet, a bell and pull, and a pot cupboard, water bottle, basin and small hanging glass'. On the walls were five prints and a painting of what the hospital would look like when finished, a drawing by Hogarth, and a clock by John Ellicott, one of the governors. A marble bust of John Harrison stood on a bracket.

As neither the West Ham Company nor the Stratford Water Company would do it cheaper, arrangements were made for water to be supplied to the hospital in Whitechapel, as it had been to the infirmary in Prescott Street, by the London Bridge and New River Water Companies. As the pressure would not be great enough to get it up to the first floor pumps for this purpose were installed in the basement. Further, as all water supply in those days was intermittent – no company guaranteed a continuous one – the committee ordered 'two Beaks, each to hold 40 Barrels' to provide against the inevitable periods when water was cut off.

Sinks had been installed outside all wards – the 'wastwater' was no longer to be flung out of the windows – but no provision had been made for sanitation for the simple reason that no adequate provision for it was possible. Plumbing was still too primitive and the water companies would never have permitted water flushing. The labourer would still have to carry buckets of soil downstairs from the privies and close-stools, the contents of which would be carried away by the night man as before or flung into the sewer running down the Mile End Road.

While these things were being done, the day when the new hospital would first open its doors was drawing nearer. At long last the order could be given 'that it be clean swept and Beds put up'. There was no formal opening but, according to the minutes, patients were admitted for the first time on 20 September 1757, 'in number thirty, they being all who offered'. This bare recital of fact suggests that there was no transfer of patients from Prescott Street, no procession of coaches and chairs carrying the sick and afflicted down the Whitechapel Road. The two hospitals ran parallel for a time as the old one emptied and the new one gradually filled. Then the former closed down, to remain a white elephant on the hands of the governors. Their landlords refused to accept surrender of their lease; they were forced to advertise, and for a long time no interest of any kind was shown in it in any quarter. Eventually they succeeded in letting it, to their immense relief, to the 'Magdalen Hospital for Penitent Prostitutes'. This had just been founded at a meeting in Batson's Coffee House in Cornhill, with Jonas Hanway, a governor of 'the London', in the chair.

The committee now turned its attention to tidying up the precincts. The Commissioners of the Middlesex and Essex turnpikes agreed to share the cost of covering up the open drain which ran down the Whitechapel Road but the committee had to build the bridge across it opposite the main entrance to the hospital. This cost £280. They also had to protect themselves against beggars. 'Ordered that the Secretary write a letter to the Keeper of White Chapel Prison that he do not suffer any begging Box to be set up either on the outside or inside of the rails at the new Hospital.' A dead-house and post-mortem room were built in the grounds at a cost of £50. Provision also had to be made for patients who died and had to be buried at the expense of the charity. So the Rev. Matthew Audley was asked 'to visit the Mount and see what was necessary to be done to fit it up for a burial place'. Part he found 'suitable for the Purpose although irregular', so this was levelled and chestnut trees planted to improve the appearance of the south front.

On 5 December 1759 the house committee 'had the pleasure of informing the General Court that the Hospital is now finished'. In so doing, of course, they referred to the centre block only. (The foundations of the wings envisaged in Mainwaring's plans had alone been dug.) They could also tell them that the hospital had been granted a charter and was now an incorporated body in law. The rules the governors had made in the conduct of their own affairs, with little modification and few additions, now had the force of law and the governors were now under statutory obligation to conform to them. They could now own land and hold property on lease. They could go to law to gain their rights in the case of a disputed will.

In the following April the governors issued their annual report. The new hospital had cost £18000. Expenditure had risen from £1146 in 1742 to £3151 in 1759–60. During the year, 1542 patients had been taken in, 354 of whom had been serious casualties and acute cases, 'received without any Recommendation whatever'. 981 had been discharged cured, 12 incurable, and 245 relieved; 135 had died, a mortality of ten per cent; 14 had been discharged 'for misbehaviour'; there were 155 in the house at the moment. 'This is the Plan of our Proceedings', they wrote, 'and though the work has been fulfilled but nineteen years, such has been the extraordinary encouragement given to it that since the

3rd of November 1740 upwards of 120,000 distressed Objects have been Relieved; and from labouring under the oppression of some of the most malignant Diseases and unhappy Accidents have been reinstated in their Honest and Industrious Capacities of Working, and so far as our observation reaches, *their Morals much amended*, whereby the Public again enjoy the Benefit of their Labour, and they and their poor Families are preserved from perishing: and prevented from being an encumbrance to the Community.'

Building the new hospital, starting from scratch and relying on voluntary contributions from day to day without a single large benefaction to back it, had been an achievement. Mr Guy had given £19000 to build his hospital and at his death left the residue of his estate, amounting to £220000, to endow it, more than enough to provide the £800 a year required to maintain it. Mr Guy's hospital had little need of voluntary subscriptions. 'The London', in consequence of lack of money, had been forced into seeking patronage and publicity from the beginning, a fact which helps to explain how it succeeded in catching up with the Westminster, not rebuilt until 1832, and its offspring St George's, not rebuilt until 1827. In spite of its humble origin in Prescott Street, 'the London', now out in the country, was almost as much in the public eye as the royal foundation of St Bartholomew's and the City's refoundation of St Thomas's in Southwark with which Mr Guy's hospital was incorporated.

The tragedy was that John Harrison, the virtual founder of 'the London', had not lived to see, what must have been his dream, come true. Sclater, Fotherley-Baker and Potter were all dead; John Snee and Shute Adams, John Harrison's great friend, were old men. Cole, the apothecary, had long since faded out. And there was one, of whom we have heard little but almost more than anyone else, John Harrison alone excepted, who deserved to live to enjoy the promised land which so much voluntary effort had created. Mrs Elizabeth Broad, elected matron in 1742, died at Prescott Street only three months before the hospital opened in Whitechapel. Again and again she must have borne the burden and heat of the crowded day. Applications for leave of absence are all recorded in the minutes and she only applied for it once! 'Mrs Broad, one of the Matrons of this Hospital, applying to the committee for Liberty to go out of Town on Thursday next, and continue there all Night, the Gentlemen agreed to the same.' That, too, was not until August 1754! No wonder that the Rev. Matthew Audley, now full-time chaplain to the hospital – he had resigned his rectorship of Rotherhithe – and destined to serve it for fifty years, thought fit to refer to 'her very great Fidelity'.

5

Adult Life

A few years after the hospital had been established in Whitechapel William Blizard entered as a dressing pupil under Henry Thompson. He had already been apprenticed to an apothecary in Mortlake and served as an assistant to a surgeon in Crutched Friars. In his spare time, too, he had attended Percival Potts' lectures on surgery at St Bartholomew's and William Saunders's lectures on chemistry at Guy's.

Now, as soon as he had completed his dressership and been admitted a member of the Surgeons' Company, he was appointed surgeon to the Magdalen Hospital in 'the London's' old premises in Prescott Street through the influence of Jonas Hanway. He also became a governor of 'the London' and in that capacity served on the house committee. In that capacity, too, he was often appointed a house visitor.

Many of the reports of these house visitors have survived. They seem to have been particularly concerned as to the spiritual welfare of patients and Blizard, a religious man, was no exception to that rule. 'Took the liberty of desiring the Nurses in the respective Wards to order a Patient who could read well to read audibly some part of the Bible to the patients at a convenient time every evening', he reported. Robert Markham was deeply concerned, 'No chaplain or prayers this day, so a dying patient was visited by myself', and later lamented how 'many patients represented to him by the nurses as being *unable* to go to chapel were really only *unwilling*'. The staff, too, were slack in this respect. 'Very few of the Household in Chapel today and of what faith they are, they would do well to consider', wrote one visitor, and another visitor was equally disturbed on this account: 'None of the Household attended Service this day'. This was too much. The committee went into action, pressure was brought to bear and a few weeks later the same visitor reported 'all the officers of the House at Chapel except the Matron'.

These reports also throw light on the conditions prevailing in the hospital round about this date. They usually found 'the House clean and in good order, the patients content with their treatment'. The state of the wards, however, was by no means always to their liking, and one gets the opinion that, in spite of the new building, standards had declined. 'No towels or soap in the women's Wards', reported one. 'The dust in George ward will soon be a great nuisance if not taken away', complained another. On one occasion 'the sink in the bleeding room was stopped up'; on another, 'all the sinks terribly out of order and no notice taken of it'. One day 'the fire in Devonshire ward was smoaking'. On another 'the wooden air flue in the kitchen had caught fire and might have had serious consequences'. And the decent disposal of the dead remained a perennial problem. Blizard 'begged leave' on one occasion 'to recommend that a Skrean be placed before the corps that are brought into the lobbies as at present they have an indelicate and rather shocking appearance'. The burial ground behind the house, too, 'had got into so improper a state', he said, 'as to be offensive to the Feelings of Humanity'.

The atmosphere of the wards was appalling. 'The west end of the Hospital', reported one visitor, 'was very offensive, so much so that I could not bear it'; Blizard himself said on one occasion that 'Devonshire smelt intolerably'. Further, the stench within must have been matched by that without. Not only had a plant been set up near by for the production of ammonia by the distillation of bones, but it was erected, we are told, 'amidst a vast assemblage of stinks: on a dunghill, adjacent to a vitriol manufactory, a bone house and lay stall [a pile of human manure], and to complete the filthy description, contiguous to a ditch full of common soil'. So runs the statement by prosecuting counsel when the governors sued Mr Minish before Lord Mansfield for creating a *public nuisance*. For, seriously worried lest the offensive nature of his works might lead to a serious depreciation of the value of their property, they had been forced into taking legal action. The staff gave unanimous evidence as to the offensive nature of the stink emanating from Mr Minish's works, but unfortunately they disagreed in public as to its noxiousness to patients. This gave the defence their chance. One witness maintained that the smell increased her appetite. Another went as far as to state that 'he could eat as good a dinner in the defendant's Laboratory as in his own Pantry, and that the smell of a ham boiling in his own Kitchen was more disagreeable than the smell at the Defendant's works'. A third made odious comparisons indeed. He said that, when he visited the wards of the hospital (which he had done pretty frequently several years past), 'the Smell of them made him sick but, when he returned home by the defendant's Works, the Smell thereof rectified him'. So the hospital lost its case.

Criticism of this kind in public had the good effect of forcing the governors into some attempt at improvement, largely due to the personal initiative of a governor. 'Mr Richard Swayne has been pleased', the house committee reported, 'to perform his Experiment of making sweet the Necessary belonging to Devonshire Ward at his own Expense which had had the desired Effect'. Indeed, it was so successful that in the autumn of 1769 contracts were signed with a plumber, carpenter and mason to convert the whole sanitary system of the hospital to this principle; references to nesessary houses and ward privies in the minutes now start to die out to be replaced by references to water closets. A system of pipes conveyed the soil down into a main drain, but there were no fixed cisterns for flushing these pipes. Water was too short for that on the first and second floors, up to which it was pumped by hand. The dirty water draining out of the sinks had to be used to flush the closets. This cannot have been efficient; nor do we know where these drains went. Repeated references to the sewer running down the Whitechapel Road, however, and the complete absence of any to cesspools under the hospital or in the garden, as at Prescott Street, suggest that they emptied into the former. It had only been covered over immediately in front of the hospital.

The recurrent drama of medical practice continued. Every now and then a pregnant woman would still have to be admitted in spite of the regulation against it. 'Last night Sarah Trigg was delivered of a boy, she being admitted under the care of Dr Leeds by the complaint of obstructions.' Epileptics continued to disturb the wards from time to time. Two women had 'terrible fits such as much disturb the rest'. Mentally deranged patients continued to get past the committee. One so ruined the peace of Sarah's that the visitor humbly recommended 'that some other place of reception more proper be found for her'. Another, out of her mind in Richmond ward, 'destrous the Curtains'. The 'distemper' of a third was, in the opinion of the visitor, 'more of idiotism than anything else as he will not take his medicines and a blister which is put on his head he immediately pulls off'. He also disturbed the ward by singing and 'therefore', continued the visitor, 'in my opinion is a very improper object for this Charity'. Infectious cases also continued to get in in spite of all precautions against it. On one occasion a venereal patient was discovered in 'the cutting ward', the special room in the attic near the theatre to which patients were sent after 'a capital operation'. Gross infestation by lice was not uncommon: John Slint, for instance, 'in want of linen from his friends, he being naked, his cloathes burnt on account of vermin'. Indeed, before long drastic action had to be taken about it. 'Ordered that one dozen thick flannel gowns be provided by the Matron; that the patients be not allowed to go to the wards until examined as to vermin, filth, etc.; that those infested be stripped in the lobbies and that their cloathes be either immersed or fumigated; the first to be done by the nurses or watches under orders from the Matron; the second by the porter under the inspection of the steward.'

The patients spat regardless. 'Ordered that a dozen coarse earthenware spitting pots be provided for each ward.' The problem of the disposal of surgical dressings had to be tackled. Three governors 'inspected the Porter's Lodge and gave directions for a proper stove to be fixed up there for burning all the Surgical

Dressings'. This done, all old dressings were 'to be immediately put into a Basket prepared for that purpose, removed by the Surgeon's Beadle, and burnt by him at the pain of his being immediately discharged'.

Discipline remained hard to maintain. On one occasion twenty patients were reported absent without leave. When one complained that another had got possession of 'his Watch, buckler and cloathes', the visitor found that they had been 'gambling, contrary to the rules of the House', but they were not discharged. Relatives and friends also often caused trouble, too many getting in in spite of a system of admission by ticket 'whereby Patients', wrote a visitor, 'in a weak and languishing condition are greatly injured, and many poor Objects interrupted while preparing themselves for their last moments'. There were so many in one ward on one occasion that he took action into his own hands. 'Sunday evening: observed many visitors that had fictitious tickets for admission from the Red Lyon Ale House [apparently they were forged and sold there, price 2d.] who were turned away by me, *Herbt. Mayo*.'

The standard of nursing had declined in the absence of the silent but firm hand of Mrs Broad. Nurse Richmond was inattentive to a patient 'because he had no money to give her'. Nurse Devonshire took 2s. out of a patient's pocket and, when asked for it back, gave him 6d. only, claiming the rest for the trouble of putting leeches on his head. Anne Dubbercombe was such 'a noisy and turbulent woman' that the visitor advised matron to discharge her immediately. Elizabeth Langston, a watch, 'was dismissed for bringing into the Ward large quantities of strong liquors for the Patients'. Before long orders had to be issued to the effect that no nurse or watch was to go out for or send for strong beer after 9 p.m. – complete prohibition only applied to spirits – and 'the door porter do not give them the keys on any account'.

Gross neglect is recorded round about this date. 'Mr Grindall was at the Hospital at ½ past six in the evening,' reported the visitor, 'where he had a patient in Richmond ward in a very dangerous state, and on whose account the most particular directions were given in the morning, but, contrary to the Rules and to every Idea of what ought to be the conduct of nurses at a Hospital, the nurse was out, and had been away the whole afternoon; and the Watcher was only there the instant of his going in. The poor fellow had not had anything given to him for a considerable time. *His life depends on the attention of the Nurses.* The Watcher found to be drunk which adds to the evil.' The writer concluded: 'for God's sake let some measures be taken to prevent this neglect. Common humanity requires this Somewhat to be done.'

Why Nurse Richmond was off duty is not recorded but there was only one nurse and one watch to each ward at this time, so the only way in which she could get off duty was to persuade the watch to stay up and take a turn of duty for her. Further, there was much sickness, not least perhaps because many of the nurses had no rooms of their own as yet (for which Mainwaring's building would provide when finished), Mr Grindall reporting 'that the lives of some of ye nurses are in danger for not having a room separate from ye ward'. There was no pool of spare nurses in those days to cope with situations of this kind, nor had holidays been dreamt of yet, although when 'on one occasion a visitor found Nurse Bowley absent from her ward' he was told by the watch who had undertaken to do her work that this 'was the usual custom on Feast day'.

These annual festivals continued to be *the* feature of the hospital year and in 1765 the Duke of York, the King's brother and the new president, signified his intention to be present. This put the committee in a flutter – it was no ordinary feast with royalty coming! Special arrangements had to be made. So they met in the Rainbow Coffee House in Cornhill, where 'the Gentlemen present agreed with Mr Oswald, the Cook, to provide for the Upper Table and 4 down the Hall (the Haberdashers'), also 2 long tables in the Parlour, and a Table in the Beadles' room for the Duke's servants'. Further, as the feast was in February and the weather cold, special arrangements had to be made for the comfort of His Royal Highness. 'Ordered that a Pot of Chocolate be ready against the Duke of York coming from the Church.'

LONDON-HOSPITAL.

THIS is to certify, that Rob.t Lloyd (Ju.Pitt) was received the 18 Day of Sept ——1750 and was discharged and return'd Thanks the 27 Day of Nov.r — 1750

JOHN LEAPIDGE, Chairman.

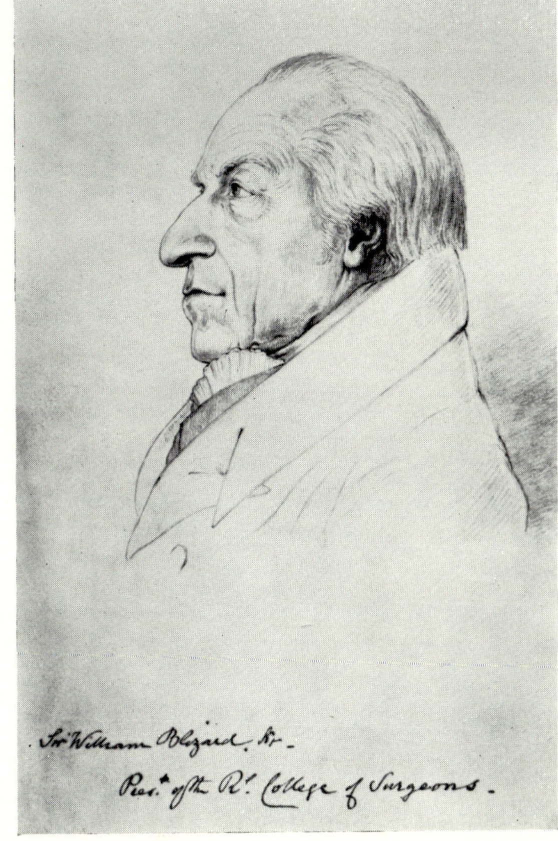

SIR WILLIAM BLIZARD
The drawing by William
Home Clift
(*Reproduced by courtesy of the
Trustees of the British
Museum*)

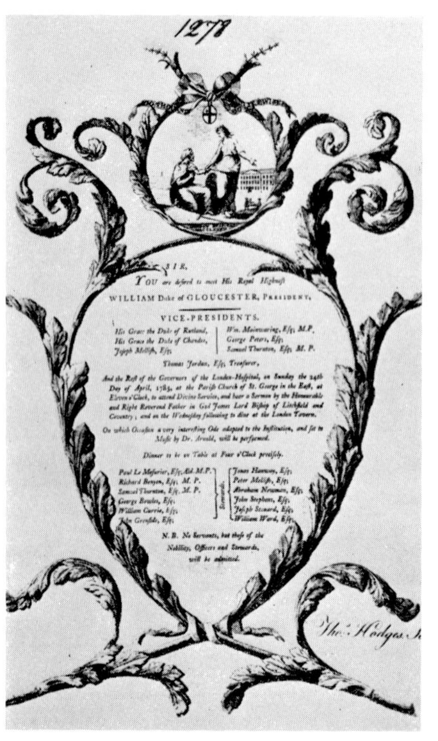

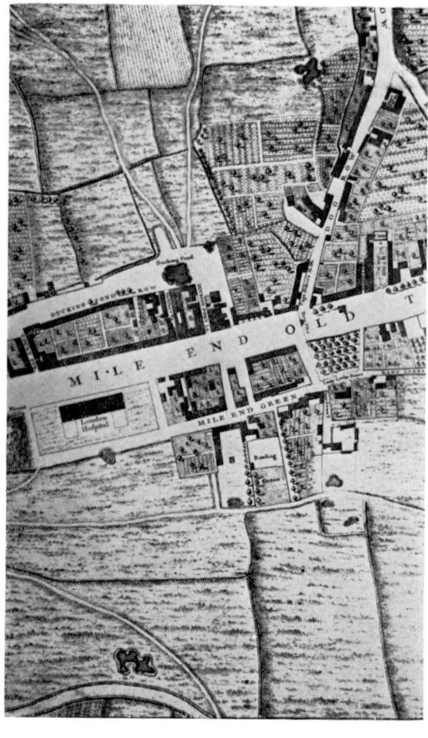

INVITATION TO A HOSPITAL
FESTIVAL

ROCQUE'S MAP OF LONDON OF 1761
SHOWING THE LONDON HOSPITAL
IN WHITECHAPEL BEFORE THE
WINGS WERE BUILT
(*Reproduced by permission of the Greater
London Council*)

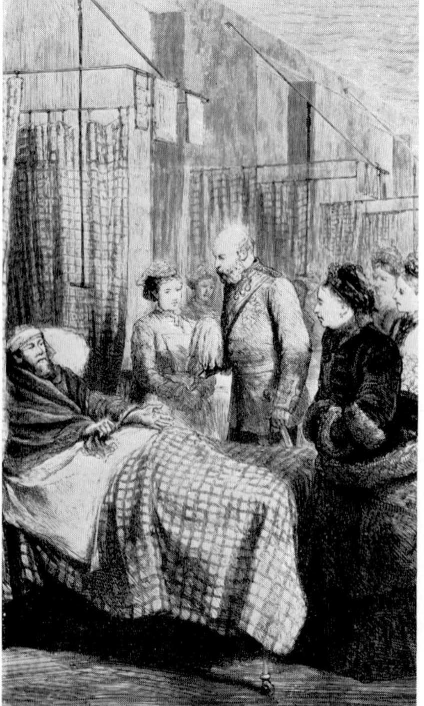

THE QUEEN IN CAMBRIDGE WARD
SPEAKING TO THOMAS CURTAIN
(*From the Graphic*)

THE OPERATING
THEATRE IN 1837

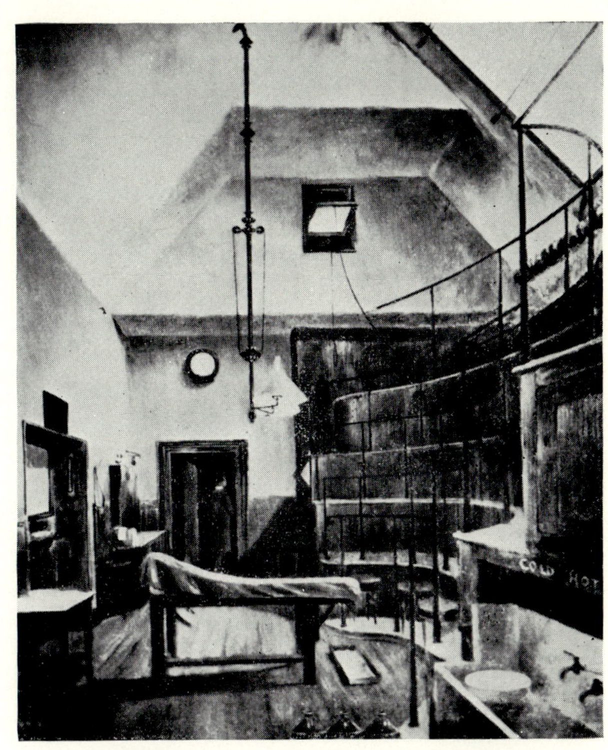

MR JONATHAN
HUTCHINSON, F.R.S.,
BY 'SPY' (LESLIE WARD)
(*From Vanity Fair 1890*)

SIR MORELL
MACKENZIE by 'Ape'
(Carlo Pellegrini)
(*From Vanity Fair 1887*)

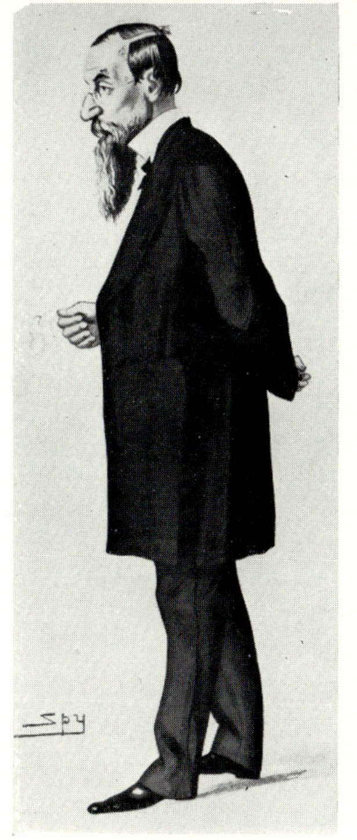

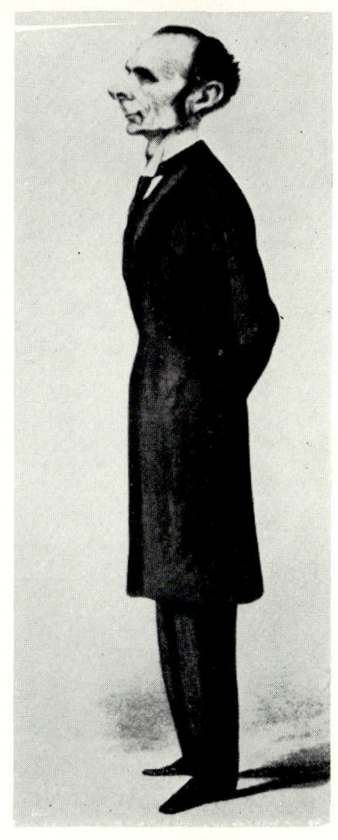

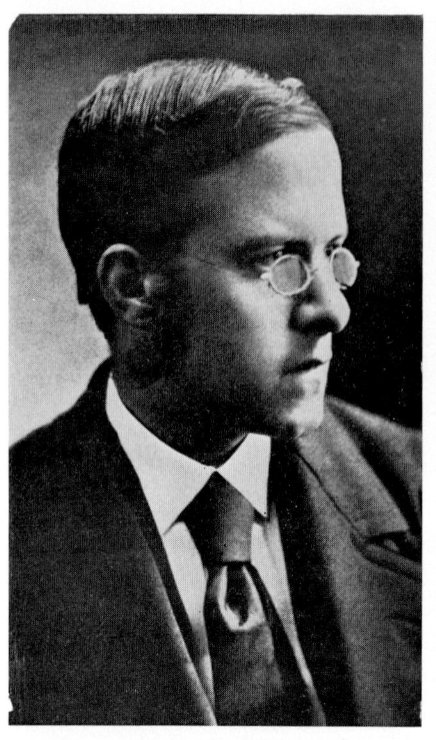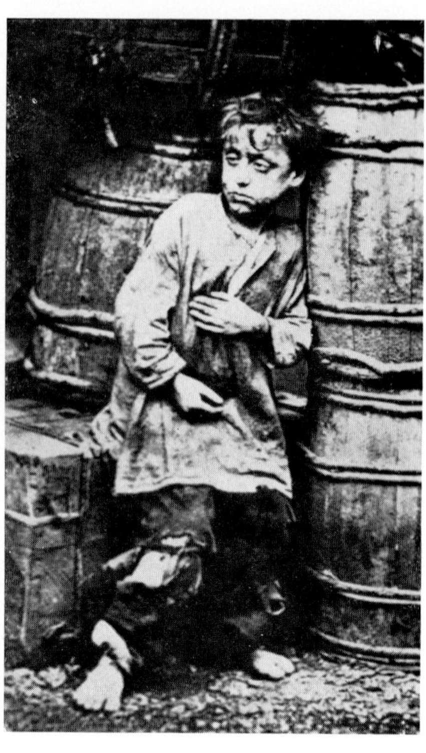

BARNARDO WHEN A STUDENT AT
THE HOSPITAL

A LONDON WAIF IN THE SIXTIES

WILFRED GRENFELL ON THE
MISSION SHIP IN THE NORTH SEA
(*Reproduced by permission of the
Grenfell Association*)

Seven years later when his brother, the Duke of Gloucester, who had succeeded him as president, attended the feast, even more elaborate arrangements were made. A deputation of gentlemen – five of them to travel in a coach and four in a chariot – were appointed to deliver dinner tickets to noblemen and the archbishops and bishops (most of whom seem to have had London addresses) living in 'the Court End of the Town' while seventy-one were delivered to important people in the City and 766 sent out by post. Among the expenses recorded for this occasion were '£3 for Wine and Cakes in the Vestry [presumably for the Lord Bishop who preached the sermon]; £5. 2s. 10d. for brandy, rum and porter'; and '£1. 7s. for heating the hall with Scotch Coals'; £130 paid to 'the Cookes' for the dinner which included, 'instead of Lobsters [apparently the usual], a proportion of Asparagus'; and £42 for 'the wines as per Mr Mondham's account'. Nevertheless, when the sixteen stewards had each stumped up their 8 guineas, they did even better than break even. They had, they found, a balance in hand of £15. 0s. 3d. This went into the poor box. Governing the London Hospital, sometimes at any rate, must have been good fun.

Meanwhile, as building and industry had been closing in on the new hospital, the demand for beds had been steadily increasing. But times were good. Britain had emerged victorious from the Seven Years' War and the financial affairs of the hospital were prospering. Subscriptions and donations continued at a high level. The East India Company sent a regular donation in recognition of the services rendered to their seamen. Mr Bowley, a vice-president, died leaving the charity £6000 in his will. So, when the committee reported 'that they were obliged to return many patients recommended by governors deem'd proper as to their Distempers for want of Room', the governors resolved (March 1770) 'that one Wing be added to the present Building, to be raised on the foundation already laid, to provide 80 Beds, according to Mr Mainwaring's original design'.

At this time, too, the hospital started to raise money by letting out on building leases some of the land which they held on long-term lease from the City, and also the agricultural land, part of the estate of the late Bailey Heath, Esq., which they had acquired in 1754. Then the unexpected happened. The other half of his estate came on the market to be sold by public auction. This was an opportunity not to be missed. The governors jumped at it and secured it for £2300, thus completing the estate of some twenty acres of which the hospital stood possessed when taken over by the state. This was destined to save the hospital from closing down when hard times came, and alone to make the modern development of the hospital possible at all.

The new wing extending out to the south was opened in 1775 and provided six new wards. They were named officially, one of them after the late vice-president who had recently left the charity that large sum of money, another after the new royal president. These now had to be furnished and the governors, after recent further trouble with bugs in the wooden bedsteads (many brought from Prescott Street), came down in favour of iron ones regardless of expense. They cost £1. 12s. apiece; with fittings £2. 15s. Each ward was also provided with a 6-foot table, two forms, a box of coals, a closet for earthenware pots, and a special locker for each patient's medicines. A sufficient number of rooms off the wards for all the nurses now seems to have been provided.

The completion of the south-east wing stimulated a start on the corresponding south-west one. We must make the building 'look symmetrical' many no doubt thought. Indeed, in the same year as the former had been begun, the quarterly court had been informed that 'several Governors and their friends are inclinable to begin the raising of a fund for completing the other wing of the Hospital on Foundations already laid'. Official permission was granted and a separate account opened. No money out of general funds, the Governors insisted, was to be spent on the new wing but such was the response that it had been completed by the end of 1778, providing six more wards furnished in the same way as those in the south-east wing. Again they were named officially; one Charlotte after the Queen and another Harrison after the virtual founder of the charity. Mainwaring's plan for the new hospital had now been completed. It had cost £23 000.

Risolière, the Huguenot refugee, had died in 1763 but, apart from that, the surgical staff had remained unchanged ever since Blizard came to the hospital in 1759. Now, in the seventies, it consisted of Richard Grindall, George Neale and Henry Thompson. Grindall, now Master of the Surgeons' Company, was well over sixty. Neale, too, was getting on in years, and Henry Thompson, John Harrison's erstwhile apprentice under whom Blizard had joined the hospital as a dresser, was doing most of the surgical work of it. Then, in 1780, Thompson himself died and a vacancy on the surgical staff was declared. Three gentlemen applied; John Andrée, old Dr Andrée's son, George Vaux and William Blizard, who was clearly by far the most outstanding. Against him stood the fact that in his early years he had been an agitator for reform. Under the pseudonym 'Curtius' he had written violent articles in the *Middlesex Chronicle of Liberty*, although since then he had changed his views and become 'a staunch supporter of Mr Pitt'. Now, at the age of thirty-seven, he had already been a governor of 'the London' for ten years and a frequent member of the house committee. He was also medical officer to the Honourable Artillery Company.

The election attracted considerable interest and there was an impressive turn-out of governors. Altogether 536 balloted, and 107 noblemen, Members of Parliament and ladies nominated governors to act as their proxies, and on counting up the votes 318 were found to have been cast for Blizard, 206 for Andrée, and 119 for Vaux. So Blizard had been elected on a split vote. His left-wing political past was not yet entirely forgotten.

Blizard's appointment to the staff gave him the opportunity for which he had long been waiting. There were already, as we have seen, a number of private medical schools in London, to one of which, it will be remembered, the surgeons at 'the London' had been caught smuggling out dead bodies for dissection. Many surgeons, too, including Blizard himself, advertised lectures in their own houses. Lectures in anatomy and surgery were also given at Surgeons' Hall. As yet, however, there was no organized medical school based on a hospital anywhere in London. To gain a complete education in medicine – and the need for that was becoming increasingly apparent – a student had to attend one of these medical schools and at the same time get taken on first as a dresser and then as a walking pupil at one of the hospitals. This involved traipsing round London – and there was no public transport in those days – which was far too time-consuming.

Blizard himself had suffered from this experience and, within a year of his election to the staff, applied to the governors for permission to give lectures in anatomy and surgery in the hospital. He got it grudgingly. On no account was he to demonstrate on hospital patients. The governors were firm about that, and Blizard realized at once that the kind of medical school he had in mind demanded its own building in which its sovereign rights could reign supreme. So, undaunted, he circulated a pamphlet entitled *On the Expediency and Utility of teaching the several branches of Physic and Surgery at the London Hospital and for creating theatres for the Purpose*. 'We are of opinion,' he wrote, 'that the teaching of the several branches of Physic and Surgery by lectures at this Hospital would prove to the credit of it.' The cost of a building for it would not exceed £600, so he and Maddocks, one of the physicians with similar ideas, requested the house committee to raise this amount of money by subscription, and, in order to encourage subscriptions, to undertake to elect any person who subscribed thirty guineas a life governor of the charity.

This revolutionary proposal met with a mixed reception. The governors had never thought seriously in terms of medical education before and their response was half-hearted. The physicians and surgeons could build what they liked, and they would let them have the bit of spare land to the east of the hospital to do it on, but on no account was expenditure on the teaching of students to get mixed up with money intended for the treatment of patients which they regarded – and rightly regarded – to be the primary object of the charity. They certainly would not agree to subscribers of thirty guineas to the school being elected life governors of the hospital. That was an absurd idea; the school must stand on its own feet. Nor would they hear of hospital patients being used for teaching. Nor were students of the school who had not been accepted by the house committee as walking pupils or dressers to be allowed inside the hospital on any pretext whatever.

Undaunted still, Blizard now issued his own appeal for funds in the form of a pamphlet: *An address to the Friends of the London Hospital and of Medical Learning*. Clinical experience was of course essential in the training of a doctor, he said, but it was not enough in itself. Knowledge of principles was also demanded. This could only be properly inculcated in students by organized lectures which must be delivered in the hospital which the student attended rather than in some place remote from it. Only in this way would practical and theoretical teaching be integrated. 'The London', he pointed out, being 'remote from places of dissapation', is an eminently suitable hospital for a medical school. 'Giving lectures would increase its fame,' he said, 'and be for the good of the patients, and the great number of gentlemen receiving their education at it, would form an attachment to it, and that, in his opinion, would greatly promote its interest.'

This appeal, backed as it was by Mr Lipstrap, chairman of the house committee at this time, proved successful, or anyhow sufficiently successful. Blizard, now a rich man as the result of a successful private practice, probably put down most of the money out of his own pocket to pay for the erection of a one-storey building providing a lecture theatre, museum, chemical laboratory and dissecting room. This was opened on 27 October 1785, an event which Blizard was always to look back upon as the greatest in his life. It was celebrated by a banquet at the Albion Tavern in Aldersgate Street. An ode to the occasion, written by Blizard – he was addicted to writing indifferent verse – and set to music by Dr Samuel Arnold, organist at Westminster Abbey, was performed by the 'Band of Musick' which Dr Arnold conducted.

Blizard is said to have been a poor lecturer. He was pompous by nature and his slow delivery no doubt rendered listening to him tedious. His real ability lay, we are told, in bedside teaching where his natural self came through. 'He was most happy,' wrote Cooke, one of his pupils and later a physician in the hospital, 'and appeared to his greatest advantage in the wards. There the aptness and vivacity of his remarks, and his ready tact in directing the attention of the students to the leading points in the cases under his care, rendered his rounds invariably instructive.' Abernethy, later surgeon to St Bartholomew's, who attended his teaching at 'the London', also tells us something about it. 'He succeeded in exciting enthusiasm in our minds', he wrote. 'I just cannot tell you how splendid and brilliant he made it all appear.' Blizard, too, had had a line from Terence inscribed on the entrance to his medical school 'in order', continued Abernethy, 'that we students should have constantly before us an admonition to Humanity drawn from a reflection of our own wants'.

Homo sum; humani nihil a me alienum puto

'I am a man and all human calamities come home to me.' At least, that was the translation (by Colman) which Blizard himself liked to adopt. This line has been the motto of the London Hospital ever since those days.

6

Through Hard Times

Early in 1782 the financial affairs of the charity came to a head. The governors suddenly discovered that they were spending far above their income. Why it was a sudden discovery is far from clear: England had already been at war with her colonies in America for some time and was now also at war with France and Spain. Prices were rising; the new wings had to be maintained. 'Coals were wasted throughout the whole House', a committee reported, 'and far too many Persons in it kept dogs'; stealing and pilfering were common they said, and the doors of the subterranean departments 'so bad as to be almost useless and to afford every opportunity for dishonest practices'.

Panic legislation followed. Governors were rationed as to the number of patients they could recommend, with admissions limited to an arbitrary twenty a week. The lay staff also fell under the axe. One of the matrons was replaced by an assistant matron at a lower salary. Money was also to be saved at the expense of the secretary and chaplain. 'Whereas the Secretary by infirmities was rendered incapable of doing the duties of his office, recommended that he be pensioned off and a new incumbent appointed who would be able to combine the duties of secretary and chaplain.'

These recommendations merely scratched the surface of the problem. Three years later the charity was still over-spending, drawing on invested capital to meet recurrent deficits in running costs, capital on which the governors had already drawn heavily in order to purchase the other half of Mr Bailey Heath's estate. In consequence of the war, too, and the uncertain political situation, the charity's holdings had all depreciated in value and were paying lower dividends. Over £11000 worth of stock had been sold and the interest on what was left was running down. 'Without a reduction of your expenditure,' said 'an extraordinary committee' of the governors, 'the Hospital will be exposed to great danger.'

The six wards in the two new wings were now shut; the number of patients in the house cut to under a hundred; one kitchen and one laundry closed. The assistant matron was given notice; the salary of the secretary-chaplain reduced to £50 and a timid court of governors, instead of cashing in on the appeal value of a hospital in debt, decreed that its annual expenditure must never exceed twice its estimated income from investments. This was fixed at £2500 per annum.

At this unhappy time John Howard, the great advocate of hospital and prison reform, was conducted round the wards by Blizard. 'This spacious building,' he wrote in a subsequent report, 'consists of 18 wards; but now seven only are occupied. There are no cisterns for water and the wards are offensive. The medical and chirurgical patients are together. I could wish there were two wards appropriated to Jew patients as they must almost starve on their scanty allowance of bread with only two pence halfpenny a day (on which Jewish patients were apparently expected to feed themselves). Perhaps proper attention to them might be repaid by subscriptions from the opulent members of their persuasion. In a dirty room in the cellar is a cold and hot bath which seems seldom used. The wards are not dirty but the House has not been white-washed for some years. Patients are generally admitted without any fee or reward to nurses, etc. Nor is any security required for expense of burial or removal. All accidents are received at any time of day or night. The patients' diet I disapprove of. The *Common Diet* is 8 oz. of meat every day [every day again which is rather surprising] for dinner; and for supper broth six days a week; no vegetables and only 12 oz. of bread a day. The breakfast every day is one pint of milk potage or water gruel; the drink 3 pints of beer in summer and 1 quart in winter. There were 120 patients in the house.'

Howard also visited the other main hospitals in London, his reports furnishing comparisons that are both interesting and odious. At the Westminster he found 71 patients in the house and at St George's 150. They paid no fees. At St Bartholomew's, where he found 428 patients, 'clean' patients paid 2s., i.e. 1s. for the sister, 6d. for the nurse and 6d. for the beadles; 'foul' (venereal) patients £1. 5s. 8d., i.e. 5s. for flannels, 6d. for the beadles, and 18s. 8d. for subsistence for two months and 2s. ward dues. Every patient, too, except in case of sudden accident, deposited 17s. 6d. against his burial expenses which was refunded to him if he had the good fortune to go out alive. At St Thomas's each one paid 3s. 6d. on admission, a 'foul' patient 10s. 6d., plus 4d. a day. All also paid the nurses for washing their linen. There were no 'water closets', Howard said, and he was 'sorry to find such great quantities of beer brought from the public houses into this and other hospitals'. Mr Guy's seems to have been more to his liking. There he was particularly impressed by the water closets. But every patient was required to put down a burial fee, this time 20s. One incident clearly got under his skin. 'To the governors, I must say, I saw a woman bring her child and with tears leave the fee of 2s. 9d. for the nurse and 6d. for the steward.'

As the result of his visit the governors of 'the London' 'exerted themselves in making several improvements in the Hospital' but, before actually doing anything, organized a surprise visit by a mixed party of lay governors and medical staff to see what really went on in the wards. As a result of this visit a number of edicts went forth. The windows of the closets were to be repaired; the east end of the building to be cleared of accumulated rubbish; all wooden bedsteads to be scrapped. The flocks in the mattresses 'was to be raked and beaten well in repeated waters in a tub by ye pump, strained and drained from the water by sieves and baskets', and spread out to dry on clean short grass. Any 'found so defiled as to be improper for further use' was to be burnt but 'none until condemned by ye Apothecary'. Medical and surgical cases were to be nursed separately in medical and surgical wards.

Shortly after this the hospital was graced by another distin-guished visitor but this time by one who had been born great rather than become great as the result of his own exertions. The president, the Duke of Gloucester, expressed his intention of coming to the hospital at the next festival and in consequence the governors decided that the bishop should preach his sermon in the hospital chapel instead of in a City church. The surveyor was consulted. Would the first floor take the weight of the hundreds of people expected to attend? Assured on that point, 'a proper pulpit made of Deal' was ordered, and a 'Purple Cloth Cushion provided for it with two worsted Topsils without fringes'. An 'appropriate anthem' was also to be 'sung, provided the proper performers can be obtained, if not, as usual by boys from the Charity School without expense'. This first royal visit to 'the London' went off without a hitch. But the president must have found his hospital in a pretty parlous state; a big modern building with a chapel that could accommodate five hundred people, but two wings out of action, all but seven wards closed, and a meagre hundred patients in the whole house.

Blizard, now doing most of the surgical work of the hospital, had long been in the habit of helping patients who had been discharged as incurable, destitute or homeless, in fact patients 'exposed to wretchedness far exceeding that of their condition when admitted', out of his own pocket. He now published a tract, *Remarks concerning Circumstances of Distress not within the Provisions of Hospitals*, and a year later followed up his words by action. Just as he had collected subscriptions to start his medical school, so he now raised the money to found a Samaritan Society, the object of which was to help patients after they had been discharged from 'the London'. This society functions to this day, its motto 'Take care of him' from the parable of the good Samaritan in St Luke's Gospel.

Under Blizard's inspiration determined effort was also made to maintain the hospital through these hard times. The medical staff endeavoured to persuade their wealthy patients to subscribe. Theatres gave charity performances in aid of it. The Drapers' Company sent an annual subscription in return for the hospital taking boys from Bancroft School, and the East India Company raised theirs. The Hudson Bay Company sent a large donation, as did too gentlemen in Madras and Bombay through an 'old Londoner' practising in the Indies. The industrial revolution was also in full swing and the population of the East End increasing, in consequence of which Mr Bailey Heath's estate, which the governors had bought nearly half a century ago, was increasing in value and was now sold up profitably on short-term building leases.

Even worse times still lay ahead. The French Revolution ran its course and in 1793 England joined the first coalition against the Republican Government of France. A bad harvest put up the price of bread and wages had to be subsidized out of the poor rate to prevent widespread starvation. The winter of 1796–7 was particularly gloomy: a mutiny at the Nore, rebellion in Ireland. Moreover, Britain was soon left to continue the war alone, the situation only saved by great naval victories. Wounded sailors were now brought into the hospital, for which the governors were paid 6d. per man a day. They also received £100 'out of the fund raised for the benefit of the Sufferers in the naval action of August last'. This was the battle of the Nile which cut off Bonaparte and his army in Egypt.

In 1800 the medical staff, fed up with the ineptitude of the governors, 'earnestly proposed that an additional ward should be opened during the winter as peculiarly distressing to the invalid poor'. So the number of beds in action was increased for a while to one hundred and fifty. Two years later the uneasy Peace of Amiens gave Napoleon the opportunity to gather his forces at Boulogne with the intention of invading England. Then war broke out again. 'Having taken into Consideration the present alarming state of the Country,' minuted the court of governors, 'we are of Opinion that it is the duty of every corporate Body to co-operate with individuals in averting the threats of our Enemies and the general exertions of the People for the protection of our King and Country.' Orders were given for the empty wards to be got ready immediately 'for such Persons as may meet with wounds or accidents in the defence of this Country, the Physicians and Surgeons having undertaken to attend such extra Patients as may be admitted under these circumstances'; that is to say, all except Blizard, who, having joined the London Military Foot Association, a body formed to support the authorities after the Gordon riots, now took command of the 6th Regiment of the London Loyal Volunteers.

For a few hectic months life at the hospital stood still. Then Napoleon, in the face of the threat to his empire from the west, broke up his camp at Boulogne and a little later Trafalgar set the seal on any attempt on his part to invade England. The country could breathe again, but the governors of the London found it increasingly difficult to make ends meet. Strict instructions were issued to effect economy. Meatless days were instituted and 'much less to be used in making broth'; no bread was to be issued until a patient had finished his previous ration; potatoes were to be used instead of bread for making poultices. (A governor also supplied beer grounds for this purpose.) Foreign wines were forbidden, and spirits and porter were only to be supplied at the express request of a member of the staff. The purchase of pewter was stopped: all utensils were to be of wood in the future. The over-seers of the poor were charged 4d. a day for every pauper ad-mitted; the government 6d. a day for every soldier and sailor; the French Consulate 2s. for every emigrée.

Despite everything the annual festival was to be held as usual, although the stewards did decide to economize by dispensing with 'vocal performers' and 'to be satisfied with the volunteer songs of the Company at large'. Only the party in the house really suffered. 'Agreed that the nurses and servants be allowed one shilling instead of the wine and veal usually given them on feast day.'

In 1806, Napoleon, having lost command of the sea, attempted to ruin Britain's trade through his 'Continental System', and conditions deteriorated further still. The hospital, it was said, became more difficult than ever to maintain, but something, one feels, had gone wrong with the administration. Could the com-mittee really not have done better? Why do we read again of wooden beds, 'very old' and 'receptacles for vermin'? Had the metal beds all been sold as scrap metal to make guns? Why were there only 130 beds in the house but 170 patients in it so that many were sleeping two in a bed, the matron again lamenting 'the blankets be so small that they scarce cover one patient'? Why were 'the necessaries attached to the wards destructive of the air necessary to health'? Why were the pipes carrying away the soil, 'depending on what water runs from the sinks', frequently obstructed and filled to overflowing? Why were the walls always damp? The minutes read like the worst days of the infirmary in Prescott Street. There must have been a reason for it, one feels, a conclusion borne out by the fact that a new house committee now came into action under the chairmanship of John Hampden Turner. This committee at once appointed two sub-committees: one to tell them how to save money and the other to tell them how to raise it.

The first of these compared the expenditure of 'the London' with that of other hospitals and 'grieved to report an apparent extravagance highly reprehensible'. There had in fact been something radically wrong with the old administration, and the new house committee now recommended securing someone thoroughly conversant with 'establishments of the Hospital kind'. This resulted in the appointment of the Reverend William Rudge as superintendent. The second committee issued an immediate appeal to the public, and raised £14000, in spite of the fact that war was raging on the Continent and Wellington's campaign in the peninsula just about to begin.

Blizard, who had done so much to help the hospital during the war, was now at the height of his reputation, one of that brilliant band who helped to make England famous as a centre of surgery in the early nineteenth century. He had done much, too, we are told, to 'elevate the surgical character'. He had been largely instrumental in founding the Royal College of Surgeons of which, in the year before Waterloo, he had been elected Master, a title later changed to that of President. Among his ceremonial duties in this capacity was that of taking over the bodies of criminals in a shed near Newgate which the college had rented because the law required these to be dissected within a certain distance of their place of execution. On these occasions Blizard was wont to wear his official robes over court dress; 'this, combined with the formality of his manner,' wrote Sir Richard Owen (often an eye-witness of the scene), 'contrasted strangely with the surly shabbiness of the hangman, the ghastly scene becoming almost ludicrous'.

A constitution of iron enabled him to combine a large private practice with scrupulous attention to his hospital duties. Only once was he seriously ill, so near dying of typhus that a number of aspiring young surgeons began to solicit the governors as his possible successor. This reached him and one of them, meeting him in Batson's coffee house later, began to mumble his apologies. 'If you can forgive me for recovering,' retorted Blizard, 'I will forgive you for soliciting.'

His practice involved him in much travelling, including long expeditions into the country, which, in those days, were often far from safe. On one occasion he was stopped by three men on the Essex road. His pistol misfired, and he was forced to give up his watch and surrender his money. On another occasion, on a night visit to the hospital to see a patient, he was kept waiting in imminent danger of assault outside its locked gates; there was no night porter then: the watches were merely instructed to go there at intervals to see if anyone wanted to get in. When he had moved from Devonshire Square to Brixton, and was travelling home late at night, he always carried a kind of broad sword in his carriage with him; with this, he once told a colleague, he 'would face the devil himself'. This time Blizard got back as good as he gave. 'Then, Sir,' came the quick retort, 'you had better see that they put it in your coffin with you!'

His interests extended far outside the hospital. Besides being surgeon to the Magdalen Hospital in Prescott Street and a member of the London Military Foot Association, he was surgeon to the Maritime School in Chelsea and to the Alms Houses for Decayed Mariners still standing in the Mile End road. With Jonas Hanway he was interested in chimney sweeps and Sunday schools. He had helped in the foundation of the Horticultural Society but later withdrew from it, thinking 'its social occasions incompatible with its scientific objects'. Blizard must have been of a little too serious a nature sometimes for ordinary human consumption.

He was strictly religious. Forms of morning and evening prayer were hung up at his suggestion beside every bed in the hospital. He insisted that the chaplain house-governor should read divine service in every ward on Sundays; a bit hard, one would have thought, on that already overworked and persevering man. It was largely due to Blizard's influence that the system by which patients gave thanks on being discharged was tightened up. The leaflet presented to each one now ran:

Through the charitable assistance of the governors of this Hospital, you have in your late affliction been provided, without any expense, with comfortable lodging and proper advice, and by the blessing of God on their human endeavours, you are now so much recovered that you will shortly be discharged. In return the Governors expect nothing from you but that you attend devoutly in chapel on Monday next, and also in your parish church on Sunday, to give thanks to God. If you were admitted on the recommendation of a Governor, you will also be given a paper to be conveyed to the Minister of your parish so that some other distressed person may now be charitably relieved.

When the invaluable Mr Rudge retired with his handsome gratuity, the office of superintendent of the hospital had been combined with that of apothecary who was now (under the Apothecaries Act passed in the year of Waterloo) entitled to practise medicine instead of, as hitherto, merely dispensing medicines prescribed by a physician. He had become a much more important person in the hospital, more like a resident medical officer today, and his work had increased accordingly. The office of secretary, recently changed in title to that of house governor, was now combined with that of chaplain in the person of the Reverend William Valentine.

His was no bed of roses. One governor complained that he neglected his spiritual responsibilities; another his lay duties; a third maintained that he had been negligent on both counts. 'The comfort of the sick and dying from the religious point of view,' said Mr Tickell, 'has not been attended to, and he has neglected

to read morning service except on Sundays.' Nor had he 'visited
the wards and all parts of the House, or properly examined the
provisions or supervized their quantity and quality, or seen that
they had been properly and economically dispersed'. The lot of
the chaplain house-governor was not a happy one. Further, while
his lay duties in connection with the administration of the hospital
increased steadily, his clerical duties continued unchanged.
'Visited all the Wards and attended Divine Service in the Chapel',
wrote one of the house visitors on a certain Sunday in March
1819, 'where a most excellent and appropriate sermon was
preached by the Rev. Will Valentine, Chaplain and House
Governor. Almost all the officers and pupils of the House were
present and with the patients the congregation amounted to more
than one hundred persons.'

Moreover, the harassed Reverend Will Valentine now became
secretary and chief almoner of Blizard's Samaritan Society.
Within two years of its foundation its thanks had already been
conveyed to Mr Blunt 'for his liberal offer of supplying glasses
for the eyes of such patients as may require them after operations'.
By 1807 they had already undertaken to supply artificial limbs to
all patients who had had amputations. Now, under Valentine's
secretaryship, it was agreed 'that some house be fixed upon
where occasional lodging can be procured for patients leaving the
Hospital unprovided with a place of residence instead of giving
them money for that purpose'. Valentine also got the society to
carry on the provision of spectacles for patients out of its general
funds. The society even went so far as to authorize him 'to engage
six beds at the Margate Sea Bathing Infirmary for the use of
patients during the ensuing season'. As 'chirurgical aids' increased
in number, they endeavoured to supply them. When, for instance, Mr John Scott reported that an artificial palate for a
patient had cost £5, they agreed to pay for it, but the case was
'not be considered as forming a precedent'.

Round about this date there were still a number of empty
rooms in the hospital; these were now allocated. One was set
aside for 'ill-conditioned sores'; another for 'states of delirium
requiring a darkened apartment and an abstraction of the causes

operating on the senses'; a third for 'cases of delicate sensibility, the recovery of which might be retarded by the laughter of the vulgar'. Specifications for new baths were approved; feather beds purchased for some cases; hair mattresses for others. A cutler was engaged to keep the surgical instruments sharp. Certain 'Gentlemen of the Jewish Nation' requested the governors to provide special accommodation for Jewish patients, but this idea had to be turned down: there were still only 240 beds in the hospital and the demand on them too great at the moment.

A determined effort was made to raise the standard of nursing. Most of the nurses, if not all, were elderly. They had already had typhus and smallpox or they could hardly have survived; as it was, the mortality among them was high. Their conduct, too, was still often far from exemplary. 'Ann Winter, a nurse in Dorriens Ward,' it was reported, 'frequently harboured her husband night and day in the said ward though he had resigned the office of Night Porter.' Nor had many of them had much education, and the committee now decided only to appoint as nurses women who could read and write; those already engaged who could not read were to be found other employment in the house. But this high standard could not be maintained; a sufficient number of women of this degree of literacy could not be found to take on the work. So the committee was forced to compromise: 'Only those nurses who could read and write were to administer medicines.' They also agreed to try to get younger women although they realized that this might cause difficulties. 'Agreed that the wages of nurses in the men's wards be higher than in women's wards, and younger nurses be hired for the women's wards and as they advance in age go from thence to men's wards, by which it is hoped that many irregularities will be prevented.'

On the recommendation of a governor to whom, we are told, 'the purposes of a Hospital rendered any measures to promote cleanliness an object of first importance', a special ward porter was now appointed. Among his duties 'was to collect all the refuse in each ward, every species of dirt from the lobbies, and report those nurses and assistant nurses [the first time we read of the

D

latter] that are negligent'. He was to carry all bandages and compresses to the wash house. 'For,' said Mr Batson, 'the order for no compresses and bandages being washed but in the wash house is neglected.' He continued: 'I have often been struck with the impropriety of plates, dishes and provisions being washed almost at the same instant as the above surgical articles.' The ward porter, he thought, 'might also scrub the new marble bath, convey the hot water to the tin ones, keep the out-patients' water closet clean, and in the absence of the Carpenter manage the warming and ventilating apparatus'. Mr Robert Batson had definite ideas on hygiene.

Meanwhile the medical school was taking shape. The pupils, as the students were still called, were now divided into surgical dressers and medical clerks. Each surgeon was allowed six of the former; each physician an unspecified number of the latter, who spent most of their time in the medical school, the teaching of medicine still being largely theoretical. The surgeons' pupils, however, attended lectures too, the committee sometimes complaining that they 'often absented themselves on the pretext of attending lectures, leaving without a proper attendant any persons brought in with Fractures and contrary to their engagement on Admission'. A senior pupil was therefore now appointed in rotation 'to hold the office of House Surgeon for three months'. His duties were clearly defined: to reside in the house; not to go out without leave; to look after the accident cases in the absence of a member of the staff; to go round the wards every morning and evening 'in order to direct and perform such offices as may be necessary'.

In 1822 this slow progress towards perfection was interrupted by another row; not between the physicians and surgeons this time – that one had blown over – but between the medical staff and the lay governors. The latter had discovered that during the previous year over three hundred non-urgent cases had been admitted without a governor's letter; a flagrant breach of the regulations which stated explicitly that, 'except in the case of acute illness and accidents, patients were only to be admitted on the recommendation of a governor and only on weekly committee days'. The governors maintained that, as they financed the charity, they alone were entitled to the right of admitting patients. The medical staff countered by pointing out that they gave their professional services free and were entitled to some reward in return. The governors retorted that they did well out of pupils' fees and private practice, and that the hospital had been founded for the benefit of 'the poor objects in the streets', not to help the better class patients of the medical staff. They dug in their heels. 'Resolved that the right of admitting patients into the Hospital remain vested solely *in the Governors thereof* through the medium of the House Committee.'

The body politic, it seems, was in a very unhealthy state round about this time. Blizard's good influence was declining. Some members of the medical staff were using their positions to further their own personal interests. Many governors were also doing precisely the same thing in their own sphere, and the cause of it largely lay in the unsatisfactory method by which elections were still being made to the medical staff, that is to say, by a ballot of the whole court of governors.

In 1807 a certain Dr Buxton who had, we are told, built up a large private practice, and had, with Dr Davies, also of 'the London' staff, founded 'the Infirmary for Asthma and Consumption' (later the Royal Chest Hospital) in City Road, was opposed by a Dr Yelloly, a Fellow of the Royal Society. The latter was the house committee's favourite but, on the day of the election, a snap decision was forced through before the ballot started to the effect that no children (by which was meant all under the age of twenty-one) were to be allowed to vote. In consequence Buxton got in. This infuriated the house committee, particularly those members of it who had deliberately made 'their children' governors in order to get their man in. They now drafted a strong protest to the court. 'Deeply impressed with the evil consequences that may result from a Law that has deprived a considerable part of the Governors of those Rights and Privileges which they had hitherto exercised – and the committee cannot but be mindful of the great benefits which have accrued from old attachments which, commencing in youth, gather in strength as they advance in age –

resolved unanimously that the late resolution of the Court, denying the right of governors under age to vote at an election, not
having been specified in the summoning for holding such a
Court, was an act illegal in itself and mischievous in its tendency,
and ought to be rescinded.' They also resolved that this resolution
should be inserted in *The Times* and *Public Ledger*, which so
alarmed the governors that they capitulated. Dr Fox had been
elected, however. Nothing could unseat him, but soon after he
resigned for 'a pecuniary consideration', presumably to help
someone else to get in, which was considered 'highly discreditable
to the profession and destructive of the best interests of this
valuable institution'.

A year later Dr Davies died and another vacancy on the staff
was advertised in the press. This time the names of the applicants
were referred to the house committee who short-listed four, two
of whom withdrew leaving Dr Little and Dr Fox to fight it out
alone. The former had suffered from infantile paralysis as a child
leaving him with a partially paralysed leg, hence his interest in
orthopaedic surgery in which he had now made a name for himself. The latter was the son of a former member of the staff who
'having accumulated a fortune fully adequate to supply his needs'
had retired before his time. This gentleman engaged a professional
canvasser to call on all governors on his behalf; so Little was
forced to do the same. Before long both were holding committee
meetings in their houses. It might have been a political election!
Dr Fox organized carriages to take his supporters to the poll;
Little was forced to do likewise. Then, on the eve of the ballot,
Fox forged a bill to the effect that Little had withdrawn from the
contest. The latter detected the trick in time. He circulated a flat
denial and was elected by a handsome majority.

The affairs of the medical school were also going far from well.
Blizard's control of it had relaxed and it had no constitution, no
rules of procedure and no governing body, with the result that the
relationship between it, as a product of private enterprise on the
part of the staff, and the hospital, which they had been primarily
elected to serve, was very far from clear. It had been built on
hospital ground and 'a proportion of the members of the staff'

now claimed that it belonged to them, in consequence of which 'various dissensions and jealousies' had arisen. A committee had been appointed to inquire into its affairs and had recommended that its management should rest in the hands of a board consisting of all members of the medical staff, any regulations they made to be subject to the approval of the house committee.

In the discussion of this report at the next court of governors the treasurer pointed out that many of the medical staff were wholly unconcerned with the medical school, and expressed the hope that the governors would always remain prepared to 'go to the ends of the earth to find the best possible men to look after the patients'. The hospital, he said, must never become a closed shop, but he saw no case for interfering with the school and moved that no action be taken on the committee's report. Mr Young, MP, on the other hand, maintained that there had been dissensions among the medical staff for years and that they were bound to continue as long as the school was allowed to remain independent of the governors of the hospital. Unless something was done in this direction, he would like to see the school closed down altogether. Here the chairman intervened. Hospital and medical school, he said, had grown up together to their common good and, whatever dissensions there might be among the medical men, these did not interfere with the services they rendered to the hospital. It could not possibly do without a medical school. With a little give and take these dissensions, which he had to admit were endangering the hospital at the moment, could be settled. Give things time to shake down. He was opposed to intervention by the court. This speech carried the day and the treasurer's resolution was now adopted. So the school was left to sort itself out without interference for the time being.

Meanwhile the governors had decided to enlarge the hospital. The need for that was urgent. An average of thirty acute medical cases and accidents were being admitted every week, and there were few beds left for patients recommended by the governors. 'Eight hundred and seventy-two persons suffering from diseases aggravated by poverty' had also been turned away during the previous year. Something had to be done and could be done about it; the odd thing was that it had not been done before. An accumulating fund, wisely started many years back to provide for expansion in the future, now stood at £25000, and the governors felt confident that an appeal to the public to enable them 'to open the doors of the Hospital to those ready to perish' would not be made in vain. Building costs, too, were low. By August 1831 the south-west wing had been extended to twice its original length, providing six new wards. The number of beds in the hospital now stood at 310.

Blizard had operated for the last time, at the age of eighty-four, amputating a leg above the knee, 'his hand', we are told, 'as steady as at any period of his life'. He was ninety when he actually retired. His services to the hospital had been tremendous: the medical school, the Samaritan Society, the medical club and, most important of all, the high standards he had set in everything he touched. He died quietly at his home in Brixton three years later in 1835.

His death marked the end of an era. It also coincided closely with the first centenary of the hospital, and the annual festival of 1840 was a major occasion. A gentleman of the Jewish persuasion promised £1000 towards the provision of special wards for 'distressed and afflicted Jews' and the collection at the church and in the hall broke all previous records. *The Lancet* waxed enthusiastic. 'Facts of this description are calculated to raise the character of the nation above all others on the face of the earth. Where beyond our shores would over £11000 be subscribed on behalf of a charity round a private dinner table?'

7

Cholera

At the turn of the first century of its existence 'the London', patronized by the aristocracy, financed and governed by the subscribers, staffed by honoraries with large and often lucrative private practices among the gentry and the *nouveau riche*, stood at the heart of a vast, built-up area. The East End had become, as the result of the expansion of London's docks and England's sea-borne trade, the most commercially important district in the whole metropolis. The iron hand of the Industrial Revolution, too, had tightened its grip on it. Heavy industry and the mass production of cheap clothing were increasing; the density of its population had mounted as the birth rate rose, cheap labour poured in from Ireland, and further waves of refugees arrived from the Continent.

These changes had started, by an accident of history, at a time when the excesses of the French Revolution had antagonized the ruling class to any change in the social order. They had continued during the period in which Britain had been fighting for her life against the new-born nationalism of France. They had occurred, too, as wealth was beginning to accumulate in the hands of a new middle class bent on getting rich quickly in the political atmosphere of *laissez-faire* but who, like the poverty-stricken men and women they employed, had no voice in the government of the country. Britain had been passing through a revolution. But her laws, the product of a happier age, remained unchanged and were now entirely unsuited to this new industrial society. Nor had any thought yet been given to the problems created by human beings crowded together in great cities.

There was no town planning. Tenements had sprung up everywhere to house workers, in spite of which many of the inhabitants of East London still had no fixed abode; almost every street had its quota of common lodging houses of varying degrees of iniquity and filth. Four out of five families lived in a single room; this served as their sleeping accommodation, kitchen and wash house, and frequently their workroom, too. The graveyards among the houses were also fast becoming as crowded as the tenements. And there was still no sanitary authority; open sewers ran down the streets. Wages were low and the corn laws kept up the price of bread. Abject poverty was rife, the hungry forties a memory for years to come. But the eighteenth-century attitude of mind persisted. The poor were always with us, the lower orders part of the structure of society and, on account of the natural tendency of man to multiply, a proportion was ever bound, it was held, to live on the verge of starvation. So, not even the evangelicals, who had liberated the slaves abroad, espoused the cause of the poor at home. There were two nations in Britain now, as Disraeli saw; the rich and the poor. Between them there was a great gulf fixed.

Poverty, squalor and insanitary conditions bred disease on a large scale. Deficiency disease was common; tuberculosis rife; accidents frequent. Typhoid was endemic due to contaminated water; typhus, on account of human infestation by lice. Then, as if all this was not enough, cholera swept across the continent from India and a river pilot picked up a vessel, said to have come from an infected port, and piloted her into Sunderland harbour. Soon after he was taken ill, and died within twenty-four hours. On the following Sunday a girl of twelve, also living on the Fish Quay, who had been well enough to go to church twice that day, was seized with 'the appalling symptoms of choleraic disease'. She died the following afternoon. On Thursday a keelman, who lived a few doors away, was found 'vomiting and purging. By the next day his condition had improved sufficiently for him to eat a mutton chop, after which he went out on the river but, on his return, was seized with rigor, cramp, vomiting and purging, and on Sunday morning was found pulseless, speaking in a husky whisper, his face livid and pinched, his limbs cramped, his purgings like meal washings'. 'This,' comments Creighton in his *History of Epidemics in Great Britain*, 'came to be regarded as the first death from Asiatic cholera in England.' On Christmas night, 1831, fifty cases were reported in Newcastle.

Cholera was a disease of which no doctors, except those who had practised in the East, had had any practical experience. 'Being in common with most of my medical Brethren,' wrote Dr Cobb, a physician to the hospital, to the house committee on 5 January, 'dissatisfied with the meagre account of the disease now so alarmingly present in Newcastle, I am induced to offer my services personally at investigating those points on which the medical reports are deficient.' The committee jumped at his offer. So Cobb booked two seats on the coach up the Great North Road, taking with him one of his clinical clerks, a young man with a paralysed leg, the same John Little who, as we have already seen, was to be elected to the staff a few years later.

Within three weeks they were back in London. Their report was alarming. This was a disease with which the hospital could not hope to cope, and the secretary was instructed to write round to all the parishes in Tower Hamlets warning that 'in the event of Cholera appearing in the Metropolis', no patients could be received into the London Hospital. Three suspicious cases were reported in Rotherhithe in February, but not until the middle of June was it raging in London, the district most affected being the riverside parishes and the City. A few cases probably died in 'the London'. The number of patients in the house rose to 323 that quarter and the mortality rate to 15 per cent. Hundreds must have been turned away.

This decision on the part of the governors may seem remiss and, to us now, look like shirking their responsibility. But the large majority of the in-patients in the hospital at this date were surgical, and it was probably realistic as, apart from opium pills, which afforded some relief, there was no treatment for cholera. Dehydration and salt depletion were not understood; antibiotics still a century away. What would have been the use of blocking beds with patients dying of cholera to the exclusion of accidents and other cases for which the surgeons could at least do something?

The pupils continued to act as house officers and in the absence of their chiefs, as members of the honorary staff were called well into my day, they carried too heavy a load of responsibility, about which the governors were beginning to be unhappy. The junior surgeon on the staff was now required to live near the hospital so as to be available in any sudden emergency; number one Mount Terrace was leased from the City for this purpose. Then they decided to replace private pupils by qualified house officers. This caused a furore. The medical staff, particularly the surgeons, rose in violent protest. The qualified man from elsewhere could not hold a candle to the average student at 'the London', they said, where the incidence of accidents was notoriously high and the opportunity to gain practical experience correspondingly great. Books were no substitute for that. Nor would it be fair to the pupils who would lose 'that personal attention to severe cases which alone gives an interest to their situation, and constitutes their sole reward for their laborious duties'. No doubt, too, the staff were influenced by considerations affecting their own pockets.

Even the pupils themselves rose in protest. 'Every one of us,' they said, 'has had the exclusive care of every patient admitted under his chief.' The new scheme would 'deprive them of that responsibility and reduce their clinical experience'. But the governors, 'although sympathetic with the aspirations of the pupils', stuck to their guns. Qualified house officers now became the rule.

In 1848 Simpson, in Edinburgh, introduced chloroform into medical practice. This was not hailed with the general enthusiasm that we are so apt to imagine. It had its dangers. The medical profession, too, is naturally conservative and this was an innovation. 'When I came to the London' – that was twelve years later – 'anaesthetics were not always used,' wrote Canon Scott, 'one of the older surgeons, going so far as to say that he "liked" to hear a good honest scream.'

The date of the first operation under chloroform at 'the London' is not recorded, the only mention of it in the minutes being when the surgeons wrote to the house committee, emphasizing the need for its administration being entrusted 'to a person conversant with the properties and effects of this important agent'. The house surgeons did not hold office long enough to gain that; the apothecary should administer it. The house committee would not have that: his duties were far too onerous already. The house surgeons, they said, must continue to give it, although they should have any special instruction which the medical staff might consider necessary.

Blizard's medical school had now become essential to, and, in that sense, an integral part of, the structure of the hospital. It had long provided the dressers. Now it furnished the house physicians, surgeons and anaesthetists and each year gold medals were awarded to those students who had exhibited 'the greatest zeal, talent and humanity'. These medals caused trouble, however, as favouritism soon became suspected. Two students wrote to *The Lancet* complaining that 'certain gentlemen were possessed of that not uncommon talent of getting into the good graces of the medical officers by their petty officiousness, seeking favouritism by undue subservience and humility'. They also pointed out that the staff were elected, 'not for their moral worth, but for their learning and ability to impart it'.

In 1851 the lecturers in the school wrote to the house committee, pointing out 'the great disadvantages under which the lecturers of the London Hospital laboured, from having to bear entirely the heavy expenses connected with the business of medical instruction'. So, when, two years later, the hospital received a bequest of £30000, the governors, bearing in mind 'the importance of well educated Pupils commensurate with the increasing requirements of the hospital,' decided that 'the present inconvenient and insufficient Buildings used as a Medical School be given up and their place supplied by one on a larger scale within the Hospital railings'. Hence a new medical college, described at an inaugural dinner as 'remarkable for the architectural taste displayed and admirable internal arrangements, the most convenient, salubrious and handsome school in the Metropolis', was opened in 1854. The senior surgeon also warmly acknowledged the liberality of the governors and expressed the gratitude of the school to the house committee which 'had so zealously promoted the erection of the new Medical College'.

In 1848 cholera broke out again, this time in a *cul-de-sac* in Whitechapel known as Hairbrain Court. This time, too, the hospital did make some attempt to cope, forced into it, perhaps, by the pressure of public opinion after the misery of the last epidemic. First the committee ordered the attics to be got ready. They were soon full. Then Richmond and Devonshire wards were also opened for cholera but, when these too were full, as they very soon were, it was decided that, as one-tenth of all the patients in the house were now cholera cases, no more of that kind should be taken in. So, of the 7000 reported cases in this second epidemic, 'the London' can again have handled only a very small proportion. For the second time the main brunt of it had fallen on the workhouses.

In 1855 cholera broke out for the third time, and after their recent experience the governors decided, as they had done in the first epidemic, against taking in any cases at all. The secretary was instructed to warn the guardians accordingly, but it proved quite impossible to implement this policy. Cholera wards had to be opened although the one-tenth rule was again applied. Again no great number of cases can have been taken in.

The idea that cholera was water-borne had now found a strong supporter. 'In explanation of the remarkable intensity of this outbreak within very definite limits,' wrote the General Board of Health, 'it has been suggested by Dr Snow that the real cause of whatever was peculiar in the case lay in the use of one particular well situate in the middle of the district and having its water contaminated by the rice-water evacuations of cholera patients. After careful enquiry we see no reason to admit this belief.' The official mind, in the absence of bacteriological knowledge, stuck to the noxious effluvia theory. But Edwin Chadwick's report on the *Sanitation of Towns* had startled the country. The importance of sanitation was coming to be realized in the sense that, if the drains did not smell and water looked clean, all was well. The great sanitary reforms of the nineteenth century were, in fact,

based on a half-truth. A commission on London drainage was
now appointed and this, in due course, recommended the construction of sewers to the sea on both sides of the river.

In spite of the cholera, many improvements both in structure
and administration had been effected in the hospital during the
last twenty years. 'Lifting machinery' had been constructed at
each end of the house; fireproof staircases and additional lavato-
ries at the end of each wing. Separate rooms had been set apart for
violent and contagious patients; the firm system introduced. Dr
Ramsbothom had been elected obstetric physician and a charity
started for poor married women residing within a mile of the hospital upon the production of a certificate of respectability. Mr
Barrett, too, had been appointed surgeon-dentist, and a senior
pupil was now detailed every three months to act as his assistant
and attend one day in every week in the dentist's room in order 'to
prevent unseemly haste in the performance of dental operations'.

A movement throughout the country for better nursing had
also been gaining ground. As early as 1840 Mrs Elizabeth Fry,
née Gurney, a Quaker family with a long association with 'the
London', had started an institute of nurses on Kaiserswerth lines.
Some of these women had come to 'the London' to gain experience. Others had gone to Guys. Later a number of sisterhoods
started within the Anglican church and as the result of Miss
Nightingale's achievements in the Crimea in 1856 nursing now
became a profession for a respectable woman at last. In 1860 the
Nightingale School of Nursing was established at St Thomas's.

The cholera epidemics had thrown an intolerable strain on the
nurses of 'the London' who, we must remember, slept in rooms
on the wards. Only the night nurses – no longer called watches –
slept out. Even in normal times, too, the strain on them must
have been almost unbearable. 'The London Hospital is the
greatest surgical institute in the metropolis,' wrote Sir John Simon,
the first MOH, in 1864, 'situated in a densely crowded district
in which the most dangerous trades are carried on and where there
is no other hospital for a very great distance.' In 1862, 4164 cases
had been admitted, one half of them accidents, and 684 'extra
cases for the preservation of life'. Admission by governor's letter

remained the rule, but less than a third of all cases had been admitted in this way.

The situation now came to a head. 'We earnestly invite the attention of the Committee,' wrote the ward visitors, 'to the duty required from the nurses who on every alternate day, after resting from 5 to 11 in the evening, then come on duty at the latter hour and remain without intermission till the same hour the following night. They are said to be frequently, as must be expected from this continuous watching, overcome with sleep.' So it is scarcely to be wondered that the matron, Mrs Nelson, who had already served the hospital for over thirty years and seen it through three cholera epidemics, had reported that 'the health of the Nurses has given way under the overwork to which they are subjected and in the absence of much larger sleeping accommodation, no further additions could be made to the Staff'. Further, not only were patients in urgent need now being turned away in large numbers, but the staff were pressing for more and more beds and special wards for this and that; for children, for ophthalmic cases, for expectant mothers, and for afflicted Jews (special accommodation for the latter had, of necessity, been allowed to lapse).

A special committee was therefore appointed under the chairmanship of Sir Fowell Buxton – the Buxton family have been intimately associated with 'the London' for generations – to consider all these problems in conjunction. 'Build', they said at once. 'Sell out stock and rely on the generosity of the public for reimbursement.' It was the only answer, and the proposal, when put to the next court of governors, was carried unanimously, £23 000 being promised at the meeting! On 4 July 1864 the foundation stone of a new west wing was laid by the Prince of Wales, later King Edward VII. Having visited several wards he 'joined a distinguished company for *déjeuner* in a large marquee after which he proposed the health of the hospital and the Princess gave formal permission for the new wing to be called after her'.

This, the Alexandra Wing (now being rebuilt on modern lines) was to have been opened by the president, the Duke of Cambridge. It was opened by cholera instead. For, early in 1866,

the disease reached London for the fourth time. Pilgrims returning from Mecca brought it to Egypt whence it was carried to
London in May, three-fourths of the cases occurring in the East
End parishes. These had not yet been connected up with the new
main drainage system.

Cases started pouring in and, within a week, the situation had
become so serious that the matron was authorized 'to employ the
largest and most efficient staff of nurses she could obtain, and to
avail herself of the services of such nursing sisters as through the
intervention of Mrs Gladstone might be procurable as supervisors
of the wards where necessary'; for Mrs Gladstone, wife of the
Chancellor of the Exchequer, was interested in the orders of
nursing sisters recently started. She had also been in the habit of
visiting the London Hospital for some years already, but Canon
Scott now wrote to stop her coming. 'I had an answer by return
of post, saying that, although she knew that her visits could be of
no direct advantage, her presence might cheer the nurses. So she
was in the cholera ward the next day, and a frequent visitor during
the whole outbreak.'

'In ten days' time we had 67 cases,' continues Canon Scott, 'and
by the end of the month 230 and 150 deaths. One laundry woman
came to work at seven but was dead by midday; and I saw two
children dead in the same bed, the second having died before
there had been time to remove the first. The mortality was so
great that Pickford's van came early every morning to remove the
dead. One morning there were forty and it was difficult to get
coffins fast enough.' Mr Nixon, house-governor, has also left an
account of the hospital at this time. 'Everywhere we had sawdust
steeped in carbolic scattered about, and under every bed there
was a large bag of it. The beds themselves were sacks of straw,
and as soon as a patient died, we carried away the bed of straw
and the sack of sawdust, to the back of the hospital, where we had
a bonfire every night.'

This, the last cholera epidemic, remains associated with the
name of Barnardo. He had just joined the college to train as a
medical missionary, and started preaching in the streets, attracting
large audiences at this time of misery and death. He also started a

ragged school in a disused donkey shed. 'There we got seats of some kind, and a crowd of idle ill-kempt youngsters filled the place as soon as the doors were open.' Soon after that, as he was shutting up one evening, he noticed a boy who showed no signs of leaving. He had no parents, no friends, no money. So, as to sleep out without visible means of support was illegal at that date, he hid night after night in some place where he was unlikely to get caught, and, bribed by a meal, he now guided Barnardo to an old clothes shop in Petticoat Lane, where there were eleven half-starved boys sleeping on a sloping roof. He pursued his researches. Hundreds of deserted children, he discovered, slept out every night like that.

The rest of his story reads like a fairy tale. One day he went to a missionary conference and gave an impromptu account of his discoveries. This was reported in the press, and a fortnight later Lord Shaftesbury asked him to dinner in Mayfair. 'Could I lead him to one of these lay-outs?' he asked. 'As soon as it is late enough,' Barnardo replied. So, shortly after midnight, cabs were called and a distinguished company set out *en route* for Queen's Shades, a *cul-de-sac* in Billingsgate. There a pile of goods was covered over tightly with tarpaulins, and, at a point where two met, Barnardo inserted a hand, grabbed an ankle and 'delivered' a ragged half-starved boy. Freedom from police intervention now having been guaranteed and a meal promised, 'the tarpaulins began to collapse for want of any boys to keep them up'. Shaftesbury turned to the student from the London Hospital. 'All London shall know about this.' And soon all London did.

DR HUGHLINGS
JACKSON, F.R.S.
The portrait by Lance
Calkin
(Reproduced by
permission of the Royal
College of Physicians)

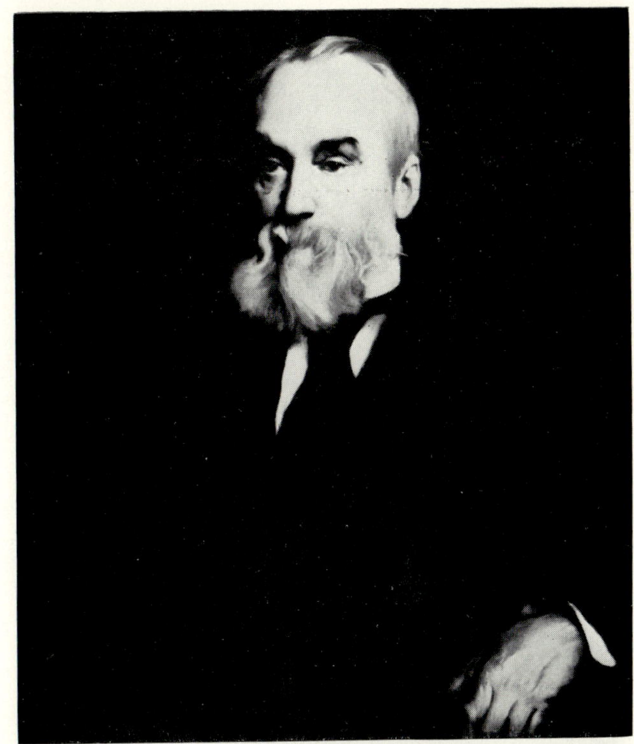

SIR FREDERICK
TREVES
The portrait by
Luke Fildes in the
Medical College

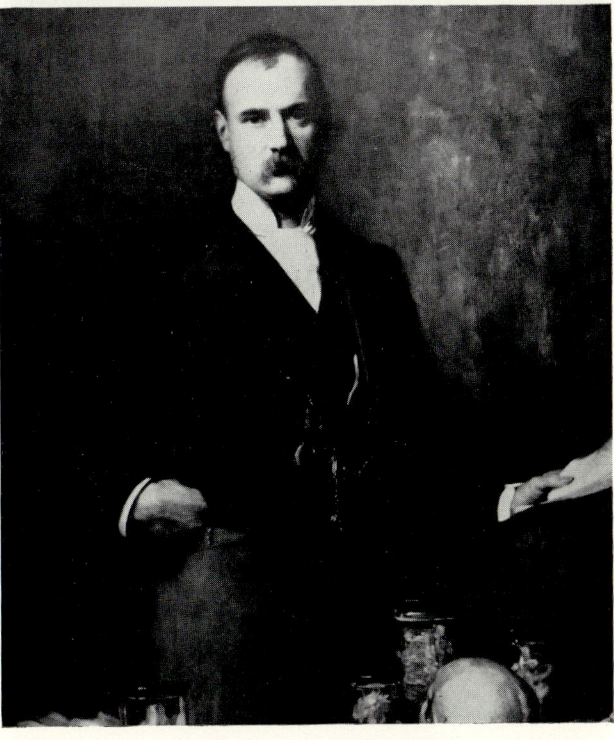

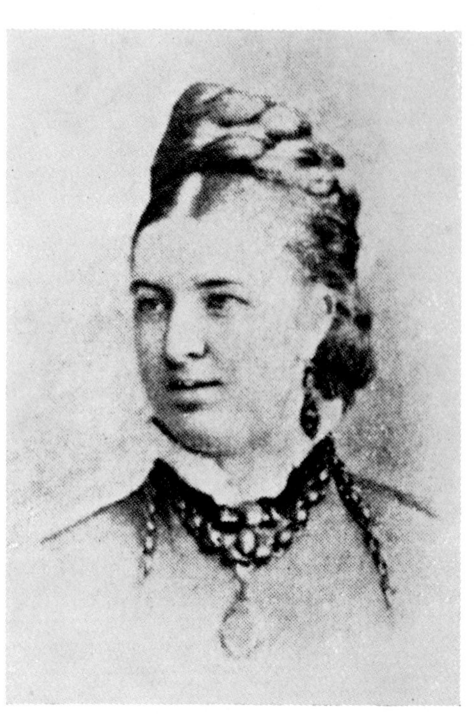

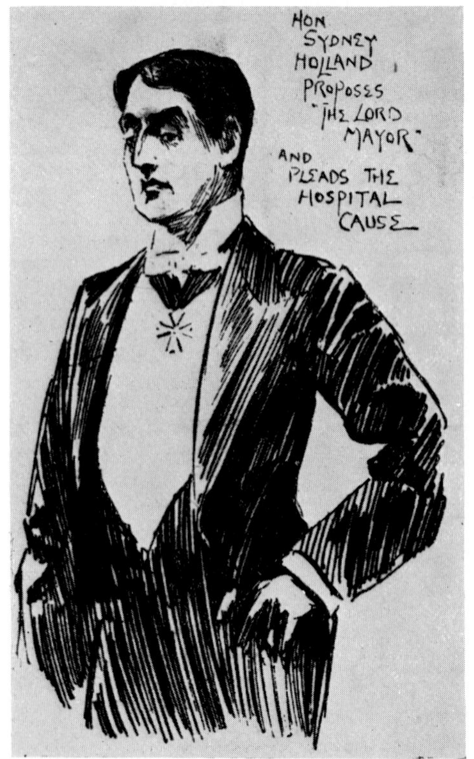

SYDNEY HOLLAND SPEAKING
(*from the Daily Telegraph*)

HARNACK, THE FIRST
X-RAY MARTYR

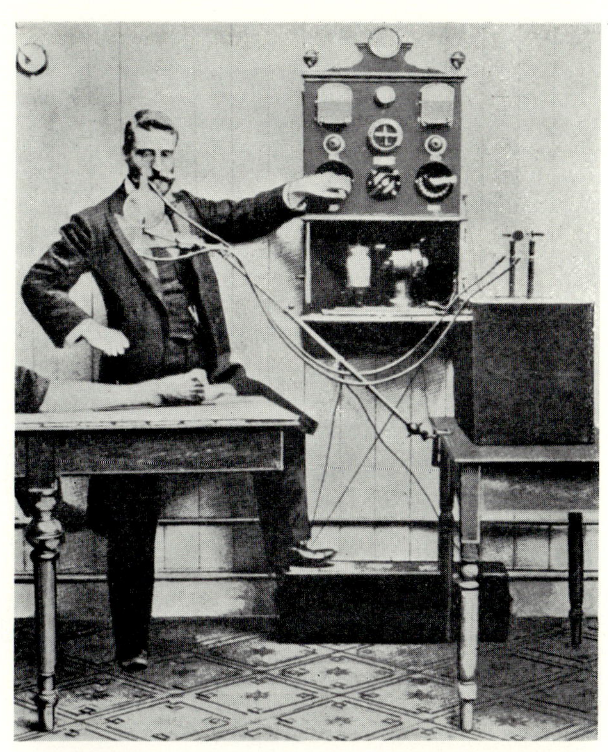

DR HEDLEY AND THE
FIRST X-RAY SET

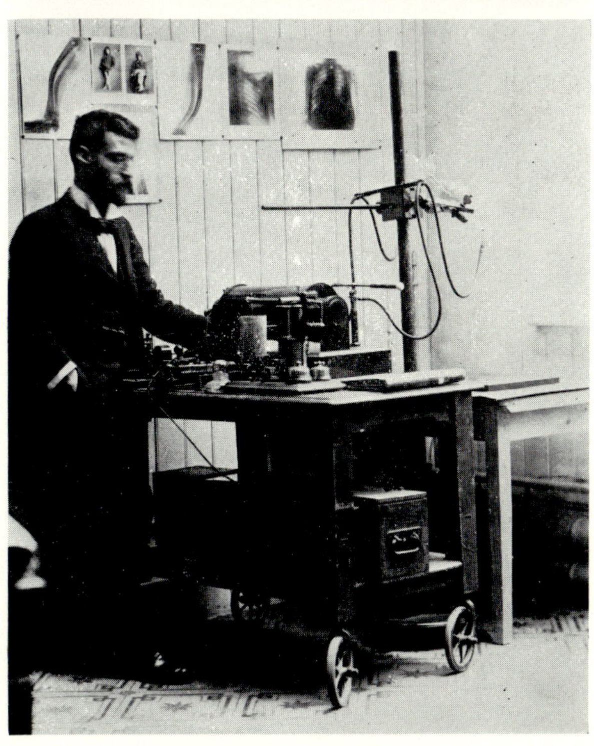

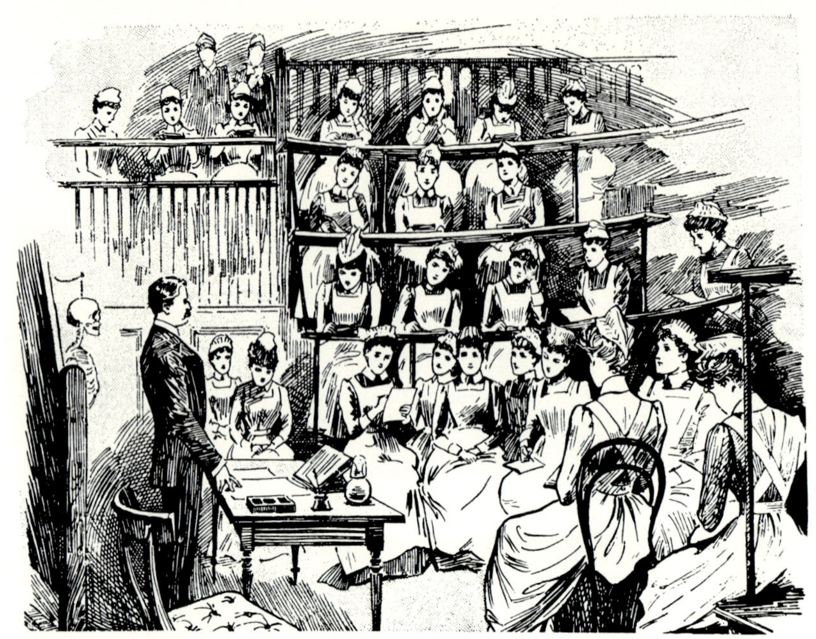

MR MANSELL MOULLIN LECTURING TO THE NURSES
(*from the Daily Graphic*)

THE NEW WING FROM THE WHITECHAPEL ROAD
(*From the Illustrated London News*)

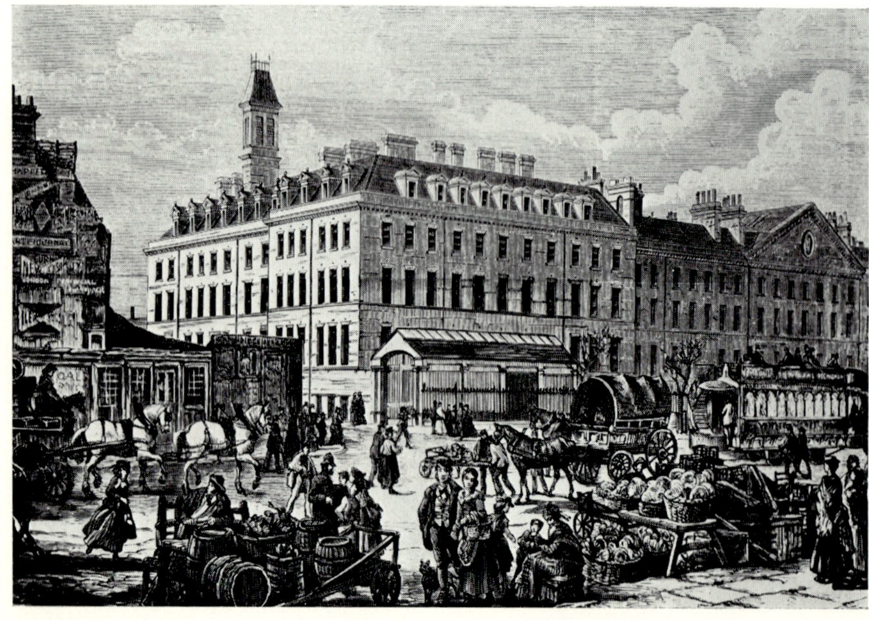

8

Towards Better Days

The completion of the Alexandra Wing permitted a number of structural alterations which had been held up by the cholera epidemics. The transfer of the administrative offices to it also allowed both considerable enlargement of the waiting hall and the construction of a new receiving room to the right of the front door as you go in.

'This was a bare hall,' wrote Treves (who joined the hospital as a student in 1867), 'provided with rows of deal benches, and there are nearly always people in it; a sniffing woman who has called for her dead husband's clothes; a breathless woman with a midwifery card; some minor accidents; a child who has swallowed a halfpenny; a serious casualty. On Saturday nights, when the atmosphere is heavy with alcohol, or on the occasion of a big dock accident, it is full of excited folk, policemen, reporters, busybodies and friends of the injured. On each side is a dressing room. The most repellent thing in it is a low sofa which has been smothered with blood and every kind of filth, and cleaned up so often that the deeply stained leather shines, and it is on this greasy black couch that the case just carried in is placed; a man ridden over in the street; a machine accident with strips of cotton shift, mangled flesh and trails of black grease; someone picked up in a lane with his throat cut; or a woman, dripping foul mud who has just been dragged out of the river.'

'This room was not always tragical like that. It might be as quiet as a room in a convent on a Sunday morning in summer, nurse sitting there on that awful sofa busy with some needlework, so placid that she might be sitting at her cottage door. She was completely without education. Yet her experience of casualties of every kind and death was vast. Further, she was entirely self-taught and of the school of Mrs Gamp, but a woman of courage and infinite resource, coarse in her language yet not unkindly in her manner, indifferent towards and skilled in, handling the drunk. She had, like most nurses of her time a leaning towards gin. But she was efficient even in her cups. The dressers regarded her with respect, and from her they learnt the elements of minor surgery and first aid.'

There were still no trained nurses in the modern sense – Miss Nightingale's school at St Thomas's had only just started – but, in the same year as Treves came to 'the London', Miss Swift succeeded Mrs Nelson as matron and she had already imbibed some of Miss Nightingale's teaching. To her must go the credit of reforming, or as I would prefer to put it, modernizing, nursing at 'the London'. It was under her matronship that, six years later, the governors decided to *establish a Nurses' Training School as a branch of the hospital*. This was first started in two houses in Philpot Street but three years later 'objections were found to an establishment of this kind being divorced from the main building in which nursing was practically learnt', and the governors decided 'to erect a new building contiguous to the S.E. Wing of the Hospital as a training school for nurses under the supervision of the Matron'.

In the same year a department of morbid anatomy was established. Post-mortems had hitherto been performed in a rather perfunctory manner by the physician who had been in charge of the patient. Andrew Clark, however, about whom more in my next chapter, took a special interest in post-mortem findings in relation to clinical diagnosis, and during the cholera epidemic he had got hold of a certain Dr Sutton to help him. So, when he became too deeply involved in practice as a physician to give much time to morbid anatomy, the work he had been doing in this field lapsed into the hands of Dr Sutton who, having now been elected an assistant physician, used his newly gained influence to persuade the governors to set aside a room in the old medical college for the microscopic examination of diseased tissue, and to build a new post-mortem room. The hospital, too, realizing the dependence of practical medicine on a good pathology service, authorized an annual grant of £300 to the department. Here Sutton continued to 'attract men to him and to his work by his magnetic personality', we are told, 'and inspired them both by his interest in and his suggestions as to theirs'.

Other special departments in the modern sense were also started round about this date. Ophthalmic beds were set apart, aural and skin clinics instituted. Structural improvements were effected in the hospital: the laundry was modernized and steam power provided; flock replaced straw in all the mattresses, renewed after the cholera epidemic, and machinery was bought for washing and drying it. Padded rooms were provided for maniacal cases – I can remember them – and better accommodation for the resident medical staff in, we are told, 'the most convenient places'. Lighting and the water supply to all parts of the hospital were both improved.

At this time, too, the hospital gave the college a helping hand. The governors had been lukewarm about Blizard's medical school in the first instance, but had now come to see the value that it would have in supplying the hospital with trained personnel and had, it will be remembered, provided the ground for, and financed the building of, the new college out of funds really intended by the donors for hospital purposes. This had been an act of great vision on their part, for which they must be given full credit. Since then the school had been able to meet its running costs and lecturers' salaries out of pupils' fees. (There was no government grant, direct or indirect, for medical education in those days.) But the staff had no capital for new development, and were now in serious need of a library and a better museum; so, the hospital lent them £2000 at 4 per cent, all obligation in respect of interest on and repayment of this loan to lapse after twenty years.

The hospital now maintained over 500 beds. It was growing fast. But East London was growing faster, its needs, as it must have seemed to the governors of that date, almost insatiable, for the

voluntary hospitals were still carrying the entire burden of the
sick poor: any part in that had been shirked by the Poor Law
Commissioners, and by the Poor Law Board which took over
from them in 1847. But the death of a pauper in Holborn Workhouse, reported in *The Lancet*, now publicized the deplorable
conditions under which many of the poor existed in these
institutions, and forced them into action. 'Workhouse management,' wrote the president of the new Poor Law Board, 'which
must be to a great degree of a deterrent character, has been
applied to the sick who are not proper objects of such a system.'
Hence, in brief, the origin, round about 1865, of the workhouse
infirmaries in the East End: Bethnal Green, Whitechapel, Mile
End, Shoreditch, St George's-in-the-East and the Bow and
Bromley Sick Asylum (all to be transferred in 1928 to the LCC
and renamed hospitals when Neville Chamberlain was Minister
of Health), with which, in the Second World War, 'the London'
was to share the dangers and to become so intimately associated.
These infirmaries now provided, under statute, for the chronic
sick, the aged and the mentally defective. A Metropolitan
Asylums Board, too, also undertook responsibility both for infectious fevers and the insane. These infirmaries, however, were
neither staffed nor equipped to deal with serious accidents and
acute illness. With this kind of thing the voluntary hospitals
were left to cope alone.

In 1867, the year after the last cholera epidemic, 'the London'
took in over two thousand accident and over a thousand acute
cases of other kinds of which less than a thousand had come in on
the recommendation of governors. All the rest had been admitted,
as we would now say, 'full duty'. The hospital was in fact dealing
almost entirely with acute sick. By 1869 total admissions had
risen to 4400; by 1871 to 4800; and now in 1872 to 5400, with
'corresponding over-crowding in the wards'. In 1867 the average
daily number of patients in the House had been 431 'with ample
space and every convenience for treatment'. Now it had risen to
516 'with serious accompanying pressure, no less than 589
patients having been on one occasion in the wards, a situation only
met by putting up extra beds'. It was becoming more and more

difficult for the medical staff ever to find a bed for a patient who was not acutely ill.

The time-honoured system of recommendation by governors' letter and actual selection for admission by the house committee – which had put the hospital on its feet in the first instance – was, in fact, breaking down, and the admission of patients was passing into the hands of the medical staff who were now forced to take them in, or to refuse them, according to their medical judgement and the bed state, at any hour of day or night. This new situation was now recognized. The old system had to go. The rule by which a governor was allowed one patient in the house at a time was rescinded and a new regulation substituted: 'each governor' – there were now nearly two thousand of them, a fact which in itself must have rendered the old system a farce – 'shall be entitled to 16 out-patient tickets per annum. In the event of a person recommended as an out-patient being deemed by the Medical Officer to require admission, he shall be admitted *if there is a bed*.'

The problem of overcrowding or turning serious accidents or the acutely ill away remained. The pressure on the beds still went on increasing, and at a time when the governors felt more than ever under a moral obligation to the district which their predecessors had undertaken to serve. So in 1873, as, in the words of the house committee, 'the actual rejection, of applicants could not be entertained in that it would have been accompanied by the daily risk of disastrous consequence', the governors decided to launch an appeal with a view to raising £10000 to supplement the income of the hospital, which was now quite inadequate to cover running costs, and at the same time to finance an extension of the hospital to the east to provide for the increased number of patients which was expected in the future. 'The London', with 800 beds, they calculated, would then have become the largest hospital in the country.

Where this vast sum of money was coming from must have seemed far from clear, but the general public seem to have been more generous than the governors of that date had dared to hope and, unbeknownst to them, a fairy godmother stood not far away. 'Resolved that a grant of £20000 pounds', read the minutes of the Grocers' Company, 'be made to the London Hospital for the purpose of erecting an East Wing, provided that the Court be entitled in perpetuity to nominate two of its members to act on the House Committee and to have six in-patient admissions at its disposal for ever.' This generous offer was at once communicated to *The Times* in a letter which continued; 'the Special Fund now being raised for extension and maintenance of the Hospital is thus brought up to £75000 [including a large sum subscribed by the Stock Exchange] and, if the various friends of the Charity will maintain their exertions, there is every reason to believe that the full amount required will be shortly obtained'.

This was over-optimistic and, of course, in those days there was no help coming from the state. The voluntary hospitals were left to fend entirely for themselves. The appeal had soon lost its initial momentum and by the end of the year fell £1000 short of the target set. The governors had however learnt at long last the appeal value of a hospital in debt. 'Risk it', they said. 'Build. That worked last time and will work again.' So plans were drawn up for a new east wing and, undaunted, the foundation stone of it was laid by the master of the Grocers' Company in June 1874, the year of the Paris Commune.

While the Grocers' Wing was being built, the pressure on the beds increased still further. In 1874 'the London' took in more patients than any other hospital in the country. Guy's took in 5040; Glasgow Royal Infirmary 5377; St Bartholomew's, 5497; 'the London', 5613, two hundred more than in 1872. A few weeks before the new wing was to be opened, too, the actual number of in-patients broke all previous records. 'The number of patients in the House, having risen this day to 641,' ran an announcement in the public press on 24 February 1876, 'notice is hereby given that, except for accidents and other cases of equal urgency, no additional accommodation can be provided in the hospital.'

The Grocers' Wing was opened by Queen Victoria in 1876. Her Majesty, wearing 'a black silk dress with a black mantle and muff to match, and a black bonnet trimmed with white flowers', drove through decorated streets in brilliant sunshine to the hospital where she was received at the gates by the Duke of

Cambridge. Thence she was conducted to a 'spacious marquee' where, after a loyal address and a number of presentations, the Home Secretary declared the new wing open. Then she expressed a wish to visit the Alexandra Wing, and was thence conducted to the children's ward where a child had confided to the chaplain that, if only she could see the Queen, she 'was sure she would get well'.

'Queen Victoria opened the Grocers' Company Wing while I was there', wrote Miss Edith Savage. 'We were told to curtsy to her, but that was all. There was nothing extra for us; not even a cake! We received a pound a month during the first year, at the end of which I was given charge of a ward with fifteen surgical beds. There was little theoretical training. We had our cubicles to sleep in but no sitting or dining room. We had two hours free once a week, and we were supposed to get an hour off every other day and a half day and a whole Sunday once a month. The nurse on night duty had four wards to look after. We had all our meals in the lobby between the wards. The daily ration consisted of an egg and half a loaf of bread; the weekly ration, half a pound of butter, half of cheese, half of sugar, and a quarter of tea. Our dinner, which came up cooked, was always meat with vegetables and milk pudding. I never saw any other pudding the whole time I was there, not even on Christmas day.'

This was the Queen's first appearance in East London since the death of the Prince Consort, and the popularity of the monarchy, regained at her accession, was still suffering from her long retirement from public life. So it was questionable how she would be received. But the crowds that turned out, and the reception accorded to her, belied all fears on this account. *The Times* waxed enthusiastic. 'English life remains an enigma to foreign critics, and the pageant yesterday, and the attitude of the people, a riddle not easily solved. Loyalty, judged by mere logic, is in modern constitutional England an impossible state of feeling. The Queen's progress yesterday was in no way comparable to a pageant of the late French Empire or to the Imperial splendour of Germany, but neither Paris nor Berlin could match the miles of streets lined with eager spectators through which the Queen passed on her way to the East End. Whitechapel and Mile End possess all the elements which in continental capitals they call the "social dangers", namely poverty, absence of the higher classes, working-class ideas. The Queen is beloved by her people, not as a benevolent despot, but as the womanly mistress of the national Household. Over and over again we have been told that this sentiment is dying out. But yet again such speculations have been refuted by facts. While the poorest and least favoured quarters of London are ready to give English Royalty such a reception, no one need be apprehensive of the "Red Spectre" in England.' Next day *Punch* came out with a cartoon depicting Her Majesty at 'the London', entitled, *Queen of the East*.

'The London', with 790 beds, was now, in the words of the house committee, 'the *largest general hospital in the United Kingdom*', and doing a corresponding amount of work. In 1877 it took in 6700 cases, a thousand more than in 1874. This included, too, over a thousand children of whom more than a hundred were under one year old. The average number of patients in the wards at any one time now was 644, as compared with 516 in 1874, a number far greater than in any other hospital in the country. Out-patients were also steadily increasing in number, and a special department for cancer and tumours, and another for diseases of the bladder, had been started. Venereal disease wards had been organized for males and females, and the attics altered to provide for noisy patients and offensive surgical cases. There were also erysipelas wards and isolation rooms for scarlet fever, diphtheria and small-pox. In 1879 the aid of the public vaccinators was invoked – at this time vaccination was done from arm to arm – and all nurses and students vaccinated.

As can be imagined, raising the necessary money to run this now vast institution remained the governors' worst headache. They cashed in, of course, on the publicity afforded by the royal opening of the Grocers' Wing. A 'Queen's Fund' had raised £24000, and this more than paid off the debt on it, but the fixed income of the charity still stood at only £14000, and the cost of running the hospital, with so many more beds in action, worked out at at least three times as much. Stock worth £21000 had to be sold out, which had reduced fixed income still further. In the following year the first quinquennial appeal in the hospital's history was launched at the Mansion House but proved only partially successful. Circumstances were inauspicious. The next appeal, that of 1883, was less successful still, raising only £61000. Only a number of legacies which fell in kept the charity solvent. Further, the People's Subscription Fund, started in 1868, by which the inhabitants of the district subscribed to their hospital, continued to bring in over £1000 a year. The Hospital Saturday Fund also cashed in on the weekly pay packet, while the Hospital Sunday Fund appealed to the general public through sermons and parish church collections.

In 1890, in spite of these perennial financial crises, a gabled front was built providing a covered way up to the front door. This, although it spoilt the aesthetic appearance of Mainwaring's original façade, provided additional floor space much needed at this time, allowing the receiving room, which Treves had described, to be enlarged and a room provided on the left, as you go in, for students waiting for their chiefs. The floor above provided a clinical theatre for lecture demonstrations. (How well I remember it and Russell Howard's demonstrations on surgical pathology in it, on Saturday mornings at 9 a.m.!) On the floor above that a new operating theatre was now constructed – but still only one – with standing room for 250 students. The attics in the roof – the clock attics – provided additional rooms for resident staff, and I well remember sleeping there when the surgical firm, on which I was a dresser, was doing its turn of 'full duty'.

The receiving room, too, was now the one that I and other 'old Londoners' remember so well, and of it, in 1896, Francis H. Low has left us his impression. 'Upon the front row of the benches sit a couple of young women scarcely more than girls, each with a child on her lap, each alike in externals and in the lack of all grace that makes womanhood attractive, and both ragged with dirty faces, seared by sickness and poverty. And yet, in the way one of them holds her child, in the softened manner in which she looks at its face and hushes its cries, there is something of womanhood and maternity; while in the other there is nothing but hard indifference and insensibility to all human feeling that extends to her child as to the rest of the universe. Close by sits another woman, still young and not uncomely, but with all hope extinguished from her face as she endeavours to support from falling the drunken companion of her misery. Side by side with a man, from whose brute-beast countenance all human qualities have been obliterated, sits a young working girl whose thin chin, moulded cheek and soft blue eyes recall the picture of a medieval painter and diffuse something of spiritual beauty round her. It is these touches that prevent the ugliness and gloom from becoming unbearable. For here, as elsewhere in life, the mixture of tragic and comic, of the debasing and the divine, are found jumbled up together.'

'Towards night time on Saturdays,' continues F. H. Low, 'the more ugly aspect of the scene becomes apparent. Wages have been paid and are being rapidly converted into the prime necessity of life to a large proportion of the surrounding population. The gin shops are crowded with boisterous men and women. This is the first act in the squalid performance. The next is blows, oaths and tears, for women play a large part in these dramas. Any weapon that comes handy serves. The next stage is the 'orspital and the victim, accompanied by a sympathetic male or female – according to sex – in a slightly less advanced condition of insobriety – walks along relating her woes at the top of her voice. Or the injury is more severe and the police ambulance has to be summoned to bring its unconscious burden to the gate of the big ugly temple of healing and death which, facing the tumultuous highway, stands dark and silent, its doors ever open and free.'

9

Eminent Victorians

The hospital was now dominated by some remarkable men; on the medical side the most outstanding were Andrew Clark and Hughlings Jackson; on the surgical, Jonathan Hutchinson and Frederick Treves; destined to influence the course of history, were Morell Mackenzie and Wilfred Grenfell.

Andrew Clark, who in his early days had taken particular interest in morbid anatomy, was now senior physician and running a fashionable practice from Cavendish Square; Gladstone and many members of the royal family were among his patients. He was also much the elder statesman, and largely responsible for putting the relationship between the hospital and the medical college on a satisfactory footing.

The former had been started by the charitable for the relief of the sick poor, the latter by a member of the medical staff in order to train doctors. Many of the governors of the hospital had been lukewarm about the latter at first. The majority, however, had soon seen the wisdom of helping the college financially as it began to repay its debts in kind. It was now providing the hospital with trained personnel and with an efficient service in respect of pathology on which, as the governors now came to realize, sound clinical medicine depended. In consequence, it was often far from clear where the responsibilities of the hospital ended and those of the college began. Again and again, too, it was doubtful who should pay for this and who should pay for that.

All these problems were now settled. The administration of the college became vested in a college board subservient to the governors of the hospital. 'We have effected,' announced Andrew Clark, 'a crucial change in the constitution of the College. Its management, hitherto conducted entirely by the Staff, has been transferred to a Board chosen in greater part from the House Committee. In fact it has been "taken over" by the hospital and in virtue of their subsidy to educational work the Governors of it will now have a ruling majority on the new College Board. To its deliberations the medical element will bring its technical knowledge, its educational experience and its high responsibility to the profession; the lay element, its larger leisure, its freedom from the disturbing influences of professional jealousy, and its moral obligations in the interests of the Hospital and the well-being of Society.'

Hughlings Jackson, Andrew Clark's younger medical colleague, was to lay the foundations of modern neurology which hitherto had been little more than an accumulation of disjointed facts. On this chaos Jackson imposed law and order. For, as Schorstein said, 'he possessed the rare gift of laborious attention to detail with the formulation of the widest generalization'.

Independently of Broca, he came to associate speech defects in right-handed people with left-sided cerebral lesions. By correlating the starting-point of convulsions with the cause of them in the individual case, as revealed by post-mortem examination, he postulated, long before it was proved experimentally, that motor departure platforms must exist in the pre-Rolandic area of the cerebral cortex. Influenced by Darwin and Herbert Spencer, he conceived of the evolution of the nervous system and of its dissolution in disease. The most recently acquired functions were, he pointed out, the first to suffer, the removal of the inhibition exercised by them on the lower centres providing the explanation of such widely different phenomena as spastic paralysis and delusions.

'I never knew him to say an unkind word to anybody,' wrote Dr F. J. Smith. 'He had the modesty which only belongs to true genius and, when we approached him with some fanciful discovery, he never made us feel small. Rather, he professed his own ignorance of the point in question, giving us the joy of believing *we* had helped him.' He loved, too, to tell stories against himself. 'Why are Dr Jackson's theories like the love of God?' Answer: 'Because they surpass all human understanding.'

'The greatest thing I have ever done was to discover Hughlings Jackson', wrote Jonathan Hutchinson, the senior member of the surgical staff. They had both been educated in the York medical school but never met until Jackson came to 'the London' in 1859 with an introduction to Hutchinson, who was also on the staff of the Royal London Ophthalmic Hospital in Moorfields and on that of the Blackfriars Hospital for Skin Diseases. He had described all the external manifestations of syphilis long before the Wasserman test! 'I do not believe in specialists,' runs the caption under his cartoon in *Vanity Fair*, 'but I believe in Mr Hutchinson because he is a specialist in everything.' Tall and stooping with a long, flowing beard he was an impressive figure, but as a teacher he was neither eloquent nor fluent, speaking hesitatingly with his eyes to the ground. Nevertheless, he made everything so interesting, and his remarks would be so fascinating and unexpected – first a reference to his own experience, then an analogy drawn from farming, then a quotation from one of the poets – that undergraduates and post-graduates flocked to all his demonstrations.

Among the more junior members of the surgical staff was Morell Mackenzie. He had already founded the Hospital for Diseases of the Throat and also the *British Journal of Laryngology*. His recently published book on diseases of the throat had been hailed as the authorative treatise on the subject with the result that when Prince Frederick of Germany (who had married Queen Victoria's eldest daughter) developed laryngeal symptoms, Mackenzie was called in consultation. Some say he was foisted on the unwilling German doctors by the Queen. Be that as it may, on arrival in Berlin he was faced with an awkward situation. They had decided to operate for what, on purely clinical grounds, they believed to be cancer of the larynx. Mackenzie protested. The risk of that operation was too great. The diagnosis must be cast-iron, he said, before they took it and, in advance of his times, advocated a biopsy. This meant getting a bit of the growth for microscopical examination, something far from easy without electrical illumination built into a laryngoscope. Mackenzie succeeded to his satisfaction, however, and when Virchow, the pathologist, could find no evidence of malignancy in it, the operation was called off. Symptomatic remedies were adopted and the Prince returned to England with Mackenzie for the celebration of Queen Victoria's Golden Jubilee.

Six months later, while the Prince was recuperating at San Remo under the care of Mark Hovell, assistant aural surgeon to 'the London' and a disciple of Mackenzie's (who had been granted special leave of absence to be with him), he developed further symptoms. Another consultation with the German doctors followed and Mackenzie now agreed that he must have cancer, and that the only hope lay in excision of his larynx. The pros and cons for this were put to the Prince. After considering the matter for some time, he decided against it. Then, the aged Emperor died and Prince Frederick ascended the throne and began to take over the affairs of state. But his breathing became obstructed; tracheotomy had to be performed, his after-care now leading to friction between Mackenzie and the German doctors who had performed it. An abscess developed in his neck and he died a few weeks later, having reigned one hundred days.

The floodgates of mutual recrimination now opened. If Mackenzie had let the German surgeons operate in the first instance, all would have been well. This was the view now held in Germany, doing a power of harm to Anglo-German relations. The German surgeons also accused Mackenzie, who had undoubtedly been right in insisting on biopsy before taking the risk of laryngectomy, of having damaged the larynx then. Mackenzie countered by accusing the German surgeons of making a false passage at tracheotomy. This, he said, had predisposed to the formation of the abscess which had determined the Prince's progressive decline. Mackenzie, too, instead of leaving the emotion engendered by this unhappy affair to cool down, rushed into print and replied to the German accusations in a book entitled *The Fatal Illness of Frederick the Noble*. This caused much hard feeling in Germany and worsened Anglo-German relations still further. Nor was it well received in this country; he had made accusations against professional colleagues, doing what they thought best, which should not be made under any circumstances whatever.

The post-mortem findings were equivocal – according to Mackenzie the German surgeons tried to keep him away from it – and the cause of the Emperor's death remains uncertain. Mackenzie himself died three years later at the age of only fifty-four. He had become a controversial figure, but it is not as an overbearing, ambitious man, and the chief actor in this unhappy affair, that we should remember him. It is as the founder of British larnygology.

Frederick Treves, who first came to the hospital as a student in 1867, was elected an assistant surgeon in 1876 and has left us an account of the hospital round about that date. Antiseptic surgery had hardly come in. 'Over the wards', he wrote, 'hung a cloud of gloom. The poor had a terror of the hospital, which was not unjustified, and many an hour I spent merely trying to persuade patients to come in for treatment. Operation results were not encouraging and the general public knew it. I remember the whole of Talbot being decimated by hospital gangrene. Every man died with the exception of two who fled the building. There was only one sponge in the ward and with that deadly instrument the nurse – who was not always sober – washed every wound in the evening using, not only the same sponge, but the same water! The fire was never allowed to go out as at any time a red-hot iron might be required to arrest bleeding. The first dressing of an amputation stump was always entrusted to the junior dresser because of the stench. Maggots in a wound were regarded as part of the normal fauna of a hospital ward and called for no particular comment.'

He also started teaching anatomy in the medical college and was naturally interested when, in 1884, one of the sordid shops immediately opposite the hospital exhibited a crude painting of a human being, with many of the characteristics of an elephant, standing against a background of palm trees. This 'elephant man', a notice said, could be seen for 2d. Treves paid his money and walked in. 'The showman pulled back the curtain,' he writes, 'revealing a bent figure, covered with a blanket and huddling over a bunsen burner trying to keep warm, which in the faint blue light seemed the embodiment of loneliness. "Stand up" called out the showman. And the thing arose slowly, letting the blanket fall. A little man, below average height, with an enormous mis-shapen head. From his forehead protruded a huge mass of bone. Another mass of bone protruded from his mouth, everting his upper lip, and it was this which had been exaggerated into an imaginary trunk. His face was as incapable of expression as a mass of gnarled wood. Never had I met such a degraded or perverted version of a human being as this lone figure displayed.'

This 'elephant man' presented a problem in diagnosis, however. Treves arranged for him to be brought across to the college for examination and, to facilitate this, gave him his visiting card, an act which was to have unforeseen consequences. He proved to be a gross case of that congenital abnormality of the development of bone and nervous tissue described by and known as Von Recklinghausen's disease.

Next day the sign over the shop had gone. The 'elephant man' disappeared. The show had been forbidden by the police, and his owner had decided to try his luck on the Continent. Before long, exhibiting him there was also forbidden, with the result that Merrick, for that was the 'elephant man's' name, had lost all value to his keeper. Anxious to get rid of him, the latter shoved him into the train at Brussels with a ticket to London. On arrival at Liverpool Street Station, mobbed by a curious crowd, he sought refuge in a waiting-room and collapsed in a corner of it.

The authorities now sought the help of the police who, finding Treves's visiting card in Merrick's pocket, sent a message to the medical college, and Treves arrived post haste. He carried him off to the hospital where, contrary to all the rules and regulations – the staff were not allowed to admit chronic cases – he put him in a single-bedded isolation ward for the night. Next day he squared the chairman who, on hearing Merrick's story, wrote an account of his life to *The Times*. Within a week money enough had been subscribed, so appealing was this letter, to endow Merrick's residence in the hospital for the rest of his natural existence, without a penny of the cost falling on its general funds.

The 'elephant man', it soon transpired, was not imbecile as Treves had thought at first. He merely shrank from people because they shrank from him, and in consequence he was, in many ways, still a child. To get over this difficulty Treves found a lady who would walk in casually, smile and shake him by the hand. This broke the ice of his social ostracism and his life soon became one long social round. Society ladies came to see him. They sent him presents. He was taken to the pantomime where he sat behind a row of hospital sisters. He spent a week in a keeper's cottage. Then his end came suddenly, much sooner than expected. One night his enormous heavy head fell forward, fracturing his spine. The 'elephant man' died in his sleep. 'He had been plunged into the Slough of Despond', wrote Treves, quoting from *Pilgrim's Progress*, 'but with many slips had gained the further shore. He had been made a spectacle in the heartless streets of Vanity Fair. He had been ill-treated, reviled and bespattered with the Mud of Disdain. But he had escaped the clutches of Giant Despair and at last reached the Place of Deliverance where his burden loosed from off his shoulders and fell from his back, so that he saw it no more.'

In 1883 Wilfred Grenfell joined the college. The office of dean (which had existed somewhat vaguely for a time) had lapsed, and discipline of a kind was maintained by an ex-naval pay-master of the name of Munro Scott. Pre-clinical and clinical courses were badly organized; many subjects were hardly taught at all, and most lectures were little more than a farce. So he had plenty of time for sport. 'I was secretary,' he writes, 'in succession of the cricket, football, and rowing clubs. I helped to move the latter from the Lea to the Thames and to start the United Hospitals Rowing Club. I rowed in the inter-hospital race two years and played in the rugger team the two years in which we won the cup. I played a few times with the United Hospitals but I found that my ways were not their ways, as I had been taught to despise alcohol and respect women.'

E

One day, when he was a 'midder boy' and returning from a maternity case through the sullen and ill-lit streets of Shadwell, he happened on a Revivalist meeting and was soon stirred by Moody's outspoken words and Sankey's hymns. He attended another meeting. This time the 'Cambridge Seven', well-known Cambridge athletes of 'muscular Christian' persuasion, were on the platform, and the speaker asked all who professed Christ to stand up. Grenfell stood up, and left feeling, in his own words, 'that he had crossed the Rubicon and must do something to prove it'. Like Barnardo before him, he now started visiting common lodging houses, forcing his way into drink shops and preaching in the streets, striving to bring the derelict humanity he saw all round him back to God. He also started a boys' club in the notorious Ratcliffe Highway leading up to St Katharine's Docks and the Tower. By getting them to take a pride in their bodies he would redeem their souls. Had he not been inspired into the Christian way of life by famous athletes himself? He also started a branch of the Boys' Brigade (founded in 1882 by Sir William Smith), and roped in Frederick Treves to help him. Both were athletes, and both had a passion for the sea. Grenfell had been brought up to sail on the estuary of the Dee. Treves held the Master Mariner's Certificate and made a rule of sailing across the Channel on Boxing Day. So, although Grenfell's record as a student was not great – Christianity and games had taken up too much of his time – when he qualified, Treves took him on as his house surgeon.

'At "the London" at that time,' Grenfell was to write later, 'everyone still worked in clouds of carbolic, and was critical of Treves who dared to discard carbolic, and was getting as good results by scrupulous attention to cleanliness alone.' Lister, who had introduced his antiseptic technique into surgery round about 1860, had already largely given up his spray and was now using heat to sterilize his instruments. Von Bergmann, too, in Berlin, who had wanted to operate on Prince Frederick, had begun to use steam to sterilize dressings. Better surgical days had in fact begun to shine. Chloroform and ether were also now used as a routine. Fewer wounds suppurated; laudable pus flowed less freely; maggots had ceased to be familiar fauna of the surgical wards.

Treves was chairman of the medical section of the *Mission to Seamen*, founded by Mather in 1882. He was now asked to find a doctor for the mission ships on the Dogger Bank. The crews of the trawlers were beset by grog ships that came out from continental ports and worked havoc among them. His choice naturally fell on Grenfell. A few years later, he responded to an appeal from Newfoundland, and he passes out of the history of 'the London' into that of his great work in Labrador.

10

Young Matron

In 1879 Miss Swift, who had been matron of the hospital for the last twelve years, and under whom the school of nursing had been started, retired. Miss Eva Lückes was appointed in her place.

Miss Swift's school, it seems, had not accomplished much. 'I had an intimate knowledge of the nursing establishment which the new Matron was now called upon to take over', Treves was to write many years later. 'Nursing was from a modern standard deplorable and from any standpoint bad; unorganized, untaught, squalid and heartless. The majority of the nurses were middle-aged or old, and a young nurse was almost unknown. The new Matron had to deal with an undisciplined company of hard-bitten veterans, who knew every trick of their poor trade, who had no inducement to take any interest in their work, and who had little character to lose. My first introduction to her was momentary. I only saw a young and pretty woman with a pleasant kindly smile. I was asked what I thought of the new Matron. I replied I could not conceive of anyone who appeared less suited to the post. I had imagined that the new Matron would be a hard-faced elderly woman with stern experience of the world and the iron bearing of a martinet. Instead, here was a young and charming lady of twenty-four whose gentle manner and quiet mien seemed more in keeping with a garden than a vast hospital in the roughest and most unsavoury part of London. I cannot imagine that a young woman, little more than a girl, was ever confronted by a position more desperate, more discouraging or indeed more hopeless. I and others prophesied disaster.'

The daughter of a country gentleman, she had had all the advantages of a Victorian lady's education; first as a 'parlour' boarder at a school in Malvern, then at Cheltenham Ladies' College, and finally at a finishing school on the Continent, soon after which her father died. For a while she had continued living at home and visiting the sick in the village. The latter had soon interested her in nursing, so she had joined the Middlesex as a lady, i.e. a paying probationer (as nurses under training were known at that time), but had had to give it up after a few months, on account of her health. Then she started again, this time at the Westminster under Miss Merryweather, one of Florence Nightingale's faithfuls. This time she completed her training and, after holding the appointment of night sister for a few months at 'the London', had become lady superintendent at the Pendlebury Children's Hospital in Manchester. There, it is said, she had had 'a difference of opinion with the governors' because, according to her arch-enemy in the years to come, Mrs Bedford Fenwick, of whom more anon, 'she had tried to establish a nursing despotism over the medical staff'. So, as the matronship of 'the London' now fell vacant, she had applied for it. Her experience was not great and many members of the house committee had thought her much too young to hold down so tough a job. Something in her personality, however, must have appealed because she was elected by a small majority over Miss Mary Pines, whose qualifications were so outstanding that she was called in and complimented on her attainments.

Miss Lückes had not been a night sister at 'the London' for nothing. She had kept her eyes open, knew in advance the situation with which she was now called upon to cope and embarked on her new responsibilities with a programme of reform which she had thought out well ahead. 'This involved no question of opportunism,' writes Treves, 'no question of merely taking advantage of such chance conditions as appeared at the moment to be favourable. Rather, she had in her mind a well-defined plan,

which she followed step by step with a firmness and persistence
that laid the foundation of her influence.'

Within twenty-four hours of taking up her duties she tackled
the house committee, now a collection of timid, middle-aged and
elderly gentlemen. Their nursing staff, she told them, was grossly
inadequate both in quality and number.

After that clear-cut beginning, recommendations followed
thick and fast. Her first recorded one is 'that lockers should be
established in the children's ward so that each one has a separate
towel and flannel instead of the same towel being used for all at
the risk of spreading contagion'. Then she engaged ward maids
'to scrub the tables and floors of the wards, bathrooms and lava-
tories and to attend to the fireplaces in order to relieve the nurses'.
This eased their burden, and before long they could be allowed
regular periods of off-duty. She also endeavoured to provide some
facilities for recreation so that, in her own words, 'the nurses
might keep their health in the service of the Charity after having
been trained in it'.

She demanded that they be better fed. When she first took over,
no breakfast was served either to the day or night staff when they
went on duty. Indeed, the only sit-down meal they ever got in
the whole twenty-four hours had been dinner at 5 p.m. The night
nurses ate and then went on duty while the day staff ate. All other
meals were simply non-existent. The nurses were issued with
rations, as Miss Savage has already reported, which they ate when
and where they could. Now, within a year of taking up her
appointment, Miss Lückes arranged for breakfast, supper and
dinner for everyone in the dining room, and also for two
separate dinners so that the night staff could have theirs at 10 a.m.
and get a bit of time off duty before they went to bed. Before
long she had taken over the catering herself.

She tackled the problem of their training which, with the
introduction of antiseptic methods, was becoming increasingly
important. In Miss Swift's days it had been entirely practical.
Now some theory was essential, and she started giving lectures to
the probationers, generally known as 'pros', her first course being
preceded by an introductory lecture by Andrew Clark to which

the house committee and medical staff were invited with their ladies. Three years later she published these lectures under the title *General Nursing*. She also started giving lectures to the sisters: *Hospital Sisters and their Duties* was incorporated in the second edition of her book. She roped in other members of the medical staff to help her. Treves started giving lectures on anatomy and surgery, a physician on physiology and medicine, and, in due course, various specialists in their own particular subjects.

Examinations for probationers were first introduced in 1882 and prizes awarded to those who gained most marks. These, and certificates for all who had reached the required standard, were presented by the Duke of Cambridge in the committee room in the presence of their friends. Before long the nurses asked for a library, so the committee authorized the matron 'to spend £6 on the purchase of books'. Then they asked for specimens, so a surgeon was asked 'to prepare a set of anatomical ones under Mr Treves' and the committee instructed the house governor 'to have a wooden case, closed with a lid, placed in the nurses' sitting-room in some place approved by the matron where these speci-mens are to be kept'. A few years later selected sisters began to help the 'pros' to prepare for their examinations. Miss Lückes would never have approved of sister tutors. 'The training of nurses must rest', she said, 'with the ward sisters who knew both them and the patients they were called upon to nurse.'

Under Miss Swift a probationer had been required to sign on for three years, at the end of which she remained under an obliga-tion to serve the hospital as a trained nurse for another year. Many women, as can be well imagined, would not commit themselves for so long a period in advance. Miss Lückes, therefore, now reduced the training period to two years, one year 'being deemed necessary', in her opinion, 'to learning the duties of a nurse'; a second as 'a test of qualification and responsibility for carrying them out in practice'. But this system did not solve the problem of recruitment. In 1884 there were still only 120 nurses, exclusive of sisters, working on the wards. As a result, the strain on them was too great, and Miss Lückes was forced to suggest that additional probationers might be recruited from among women who could afford to pay, as was already being done at other hospitals. If this scheme was to work, however, better living accommodation would have to be found, 'as some of them would be ladies and paying probationers would not long dispense with the amenities of a single bedroom'. Again the committee accepted her recommendations and an advertisement to this effect was inserted in *The Guardian* and *The Queen*. Before long we find her asking for 'a special bathroom for the night nurses as the better class of woman now engaged made rather a point of conveniences for personal cleanliness'.

Inadequate accommodation for her staff remained the great barrier to any real improvement in the standard of life of her nurses. This was the desperate, almost heart-breaking handicap with which the new young matron had to contend. Until she got more accommodation, how could she engage more nurses? Until she got more nurses, how could she reduce the hours that they had to work? Until their work was reduced, what hope was there of training them better? Until their living accommodation was improved, what chance was there of getting a better class of woman to apply? It was a terrible impasse. The truth was that during the past few years the hospital had, as the result of the ever-increasing demand on its services, long since passed the point when it could still nurse its patients properly. Its whole future now depended on the provision of better accommodation for the nursing staff. So, again and again we find Miss Lückes pressing the house committee to do something about it, pointing out the impossibility of maintaining standards when, in her own words, 'the bedrooms of her nurses were scattered in five directions'. Sisters still slept in rooms between the wards. Some of the night and day staff 'boxed and coxed' in the attics of the Grocers' wing, others in odd rooms scattered round the hospital or in hired ones out on the estate. A few lived at home and came in daily. Night nurses were even sometimes hired at this time from among the women who gathered in the hall each evening to offer their services in some menial capacity.

For the moment, with the best will in the world, the house

committee could do nothing to help her. The funds of the hospital would simply not permit. Then, in the autumn of 1884, came the stroke of luck which she had so richly deserved. The East London Railway wanted to extend their line from Whitechapel to Surrey Docks and now sought the right to carry a line under the hospital estate with a view to the construction of a tunnel under the river by the famous engineer Brunel. The governors, in a strong position, sold this for £30000 and decided to devote the greater part of it at once to building a home to provide separate rooms for at least a hundred nurses.

Meanwhile, as the nursing school had been taking shape, the medical college had yet again begun to outgrow its habitation. The staff of the hospital was distinguished, and the East End now provided an opportunity to gain clinical experience unrivalled in the rest of London. What was to be done? Add on to the already patchwork building or take the bull by the horns and rebuild completely? The matter was discussed at length and eventually the board of the college decided to ask the governors of the hospital for a loan of £15000. The relationships between hospital and college were now happier than at any previous period in the latter's history. The 'Act of Union' (when the college board first came into being) had been an outstanding success. The request was granted. So two new buildings were now rising simultaneously; a new nurses' home at the southern end of the east wing, and, to all intents and purposes, a new college where the college stands today.

Both buildings were opened by the Prince and Princess of Wales in May 1877. 'After a formal reception at the main gate,' wrote *The Times*, 'the Royal party visited a number of wards and then proceeded to the new Home where they were received by the Matron at the head of the nursing staff in their plain but tasteful uniform of print gown and white mob cap and apron. The Princess formally declared the Alexandra Home open. Then the procession moved through the garden to the Medical College, whence it was conducted to the new library where 300 people were assembled and a dais had been erected at one end.' The Prince now made a speech in which he referred to the hospital as having undertaken the difficult task of providing a higher class of nursing staff with better discipline and superior training, and also to the new library and building, which he was about to declare open, as 'belonging to a College over a hundred years old, the first in which a complete medical curriculum had been established and now belonging to the largest hospital in the country'.

Blizard had founded the medical college nearly a hundred years ago. Miss Lückes had now put the nursing school on its feet. 'We did not know', wrote Treves – he was looking back to the day on which she had been appointed – 'that we had to deal with one of the ablest and most remarkable women of the age, an organizer with unequalled genius, with the tact and foresight of a diplomat, and the imagination of a maker of new worlds. Nor did we realize that beneath that pleasing and gentle manner was a determination and a will that could be daunted by no difficulty nor turned aside by any obstacle. How this amazing woman accomplished the feat I do not know. But I do know that slowly and quietly, without friction, without disturbance and without rows, the Hospital had become transformed. There breathed through the harsh and dismal building a woman's influence like a breath of Spring. By some magic force the nurses became obedient, efficient and proud of their work.'

I I

Before the Lords

When Miss Lückes took up her matronship at 'the London' the voluntary hospitals were no longer the only hospitals in the metropolis. The poor law or workhouse infirmaries were also now well established.

The former had been started by private enterprise to meet a social need. The bases of the medical and nursing schools (also begun by individual effort), they had set the pace and made the running in respect of the standard of medical practice. But their existence was precarious; they depended entirely on voluntary contribution. The latter had been started by the state in order to bridge the widening gap in the provision of medical care for the sick poor as the population of London increased, and were under a statutory obligation to take the aged and other chronic sick with which the voluntary hospitals could not afford to block their beds. They were maintained, as frugally as possible, out of the rates. The voluntaries dealt with all the serious accidents and with most acute illness, for which the infirmaries were neither staffed nor equipped to cope, and unloaded their semi-convalescents and failures, and all the patients for whom they could do nothing, on to the workhouse infirmaries.

The organization of the hospitals in the metropolis was in fact chaotic, not on account of mistaken legislation, but by reason of the unplanned manner in which it had evolved. Criticism of it had now become outspoken both in the medical and lay press. The poor-law infirmaries, largely out of sight and well out of public mind, prison-like outside and Dickensian within, escaped most of it. Not so the voluntary hospitals. Patronized by royalty and the aristocracy, well before the public in consequence of their appeals for more and more money to help them to soldier on, they had become fair game. Some said they were drifting into chronic bankruptcy because they insisted on sticking to the ridiculous policy of providing for one class only, namely the necessitous poor. Why not start pay wards? Others maintained that they were encouraging the working class to depend on charity. If they could afford to get drunk, they could afford to pay when they got ill. Some said that pride stopped many going into hospital where they would be compelled to accept charity. Others pointed to the waste of all those competitive appeals of which the general public were getting heartily tired. The voluntary hospitals, too, might be centres of excellence, but to many they were also islands of privilege. It was necessary, some said, for the poor man to know the right governor, or go to the right doctor, to wangle himself in as a patient. What was needed, said many, was a central health authority.

The matter came to a head in the tenth year of Miss Lückes's matronship when Lord Sandhurst, in response to a petition from the Charity Organization Society (which offered a possible alternative to the future Welfare State), moved for the setting up of a Select Committee of the House of Lords to inquire into the working of the metropolitan hospitals in general. This was a highly laudable idea – something of the kind was already long overdue – but it seems to have been used by, and possibly even to have been instigated at the suggestion of, a group within the Society who were also governors of 'the London', and, although in a minority, had a particular grouse against 'the London' and against its matron in particular.

This disgruntled minority consisted of a Mr Yatman, whose daughter had been a probationer under Miss Lückes; Mr and Mrs Hall, friends of the Yatmans; and Mrs Bedford Fenwick. The latter was the daughter-in-law of Dr Fenwick, now physician in charge of the nurses. Her husband had failed to get elected to 'the London' staff like his father and, having been in love with Miss

Lückes (according to current gossip), had ended by marrying Miss Manton, the matron of Bart's. This lady, now Mrs Bedford Fenwick, was the same age as Miss Lückes and had also been a sister at 'the London', but had not applied for the matronship when Miss Lückes was appointed, probably because she knew she would not get it. Now she had elected to champion the cause of nurses in general. She had founded the British Nursing Association, and gained control of the *Nursing Record*, the only journal devoted exclusively to nursing at that date. She had also started to fight for the state recognition of nurses, something to which Miss Nightingale and Miss Lückes, who believed in competition and individual hospital certificates, were both hotly opposed. 'State registration', said Miss Lückes, 'would standardize mediocrity.'

After a preliminary meeting of the Select Committee, at which members of the COS were questioned and it must have been decided to take 'the London' before all the other hospitals, certain ex-members of the nursing staff were called before them to give evidence. How these witnesses were selected is far from clear. Indeed, it looks very much as if they selected themselves in the sense that they volunteered to come. What is clear is that, whatever may have been the motive of the Society in getting the Select Committee set up, it now provided a forum for an all-out attack on 'the London'. Its meetings were fully reported in the press.

Miss Yatman said she had been overworked and underfed and had had an attack of blood poisoning due to an escape of sewer gas. Again and again, she went on, nurses were compelled to work when they were ill; Miss Lambert, for example, had had to go on duty with scarlet fever; Miss Scott and Miss Furnace with poisoned hands. Miss Sable had died from a poisoned finger and a sore throat. Asked about the food, she said that their only substantial meal was dinner; at other times only potted lobster, sardines and pickled mackerel. The night nurses would often go on duty with nothing but half a herring and a bun! Probationers who paid the hospital £20 a year, she said, were sent out to private cases who paid the hospital £2 a week and thought they were getting trained nurses for their money! Lord Kimberley: 'Then the advertisement put out is not only fraudulent, but money is actually received on false pretences?' Miss Yatman: 'Yes.'

Miss Raymond confirmed what Miss Yatman had said and made accusations of her own. In a children's ward with fifty-six cots there were only three nurses! In another ward a patient, after an anaesthetic, fell out of bed because no nurse could be spared to watch him. She agreed that their health was neglected. They were also insufficiently protected from the matron who had dismissed her just because she went to see her own doctor! If they complained about anything they were dismissed at once, and so on and so on.

Then a former chaplain, who 'had thought it his duty to bring many grave abuses to the attention of the House Committee', was called. (He may have offered to come.) There were not enough qualified nurses, he said, and far too many paying probationers. The conditions, too, under which they lived were deplorable. 'Through the cracks and crannies of the Sisters' rooms crept the stench of gangrene and cancer.' Further, 'the Matron had established a petty tyranny and the nurses were all afraid to complain'. As one member of the committee had said to another, 'We are all under petticoat government now!'

The chairman countered their accusations vigorously but was forced to admit that absolute power of dismissing probationers had been delegated to the matron, although all had had the right of appeal to the house committee. In the last ten years only eight out of six hundred had, in fact, been dismissed. Questioned about the chaplain, he said that he had no specific charges to make against him, but he had grown out of accord with the committee and was very high church. He, the chaplain, had since told him that he 'would not leave a stone unturned to do the Hospital injury'.

Miss Lückes gave evidence on four occasions, in one of which she was in the 'witness box' all day. Asked about her staff, she told the committee that she had one nurse to every $3\frac{1}{2}$ patients, as opposed to one in five when she was first appointed. Questioned about their working hours, she said that the day nurses did fourteen hours on duty, with two hours off, and the night nurses twelve. Days off, she had to admit, were few and far between. Lord Thring: 'Do you not think a fourteen-hour day every day of the week too much for an ordinary woman?' Her reply was significant. 'I do not think a nurse is an ordinary woman or she would not have taken up nursing.' Lord Thring: 'Would it be too much for an *ordinary* woman?' Her reply was categorical: 'If her health was good she would not suffer.' If, however, economy in administration had not been necessary, she went on, she would have 'liked to see nurses' working hours shortened, their holidays lengthened and their pay increased, as the three legitimate means by which nursing could be advanced'.

The feeding of her nurses, she maintained, had been considerably improved since she took over the catering. All now had sit-down meals before going on and also after coming off duty. The drains had caused trouble but this had now been put right; the sewer gas, of which Miss Yatman had complained, was ordinary coal gas. Miss Lambert, it is true, had been sent on duty with scarlet fever, which she much regretted, but she had letters from Miss Scott and Miss Furnace denying that they had ever been made to work with septic hands, as had been alleged by Miss Yatman. Miss Sable, too, had not died from a poisoned finger, as Miss Yatman had also said, but from diphtheria contracted while nursing a private patient. Dr Fenwick and Dr Sutton, she said, were in the hospital every day to see any nurse who wanted to consult them; Mr Treves was always called when surgical advice was required. Every precaution was taken to ensure her nurses' good health. There had been fifteen deaths among them, it was true, in the last ten years, but the sickness rate was not unduly high and what sickness there was could not be attributed to overwork.

Dr Fenwick corroborated everything that Miss Lückes had said and had nothing but praise for the work of the nurses. He admitted that they worked hard and, even more vigorously than Miss Lückes herself, stressed the need for shorter hours and longer holidays as soon as economic factors would allow it.

For the young matron – she was still only thirty-four – loyally though she had been backed by the house committee and the

medical staff, it had been, to use her own words, 'a time of pur-
gatory'. Not only did she have to face the Lords day after day
but every night she had had to read the garbled accounts of
'scandals' at 'the London' which appeared every day in the public
press. 'Day after day letters, wild suggestions, telegrams, keep
pouring in', she wrote to Miss Nightingale. 'You will know how
deeply I have been moved all along by these troubles', the latter
replied, 'and I pray for all the blessings of the New Year that
Infinite Love can give to one who has fought so well. Everything
will turn out right. You have made an army of friends.'

Certain sections of the press were scathing. *The Charity Record*
came out with an article entitled 'The Trial of the London
Hospital'. *The East London Advertiser* was peculiarly hostile, but
the most virulent articles appeared in Mrs Bedford Fenwick's
Nursing Record in which she made full use of the 'scandals' at the
London Hospital as ammunition with which to further her campaign for the state registration of nurses. 'There is no disguising
the fact', ran a clearly inspired editorial, 'that the London Hospital has now for some time past turned out annually an ever
increasing number of young ladies with an amateur smattering
of the rudiments of nursing gained in a three months' course as
paying probationers.'

The *Pall Mall Gazette* endeavoured to be fair. First it published
a long article, 'Does the London Hospital sweat its nurses? An
Interview with Mrs Hunter', and then followed this up with, 'No,
not much more than others. An Interview with Miss Walker'.
The Hospital came down more definitely still on 'the London's'
side. 'It has been affirmed on one side', the editor wrote, 'that a
dead-set has been made against "the London" by an organized
opposition but the whole accusation amounts to no more than
this: that at some recent period certain nurses were overworked
and that they were not delicately fed. And it is not proved to be
true. On the contrary, the weight of responsible evidence leads
to the conclusion that the nurses at the London Hospital are as
liberally fed and as reasonably worked as nurses can expect at an
institution of that kind.'

The evidence given before the Lords was debated by the

SYDNEY HOLLAND, SECOND VISCOUNT KNUTSFORD
The portrait by Oswald Birley at the London Hospital

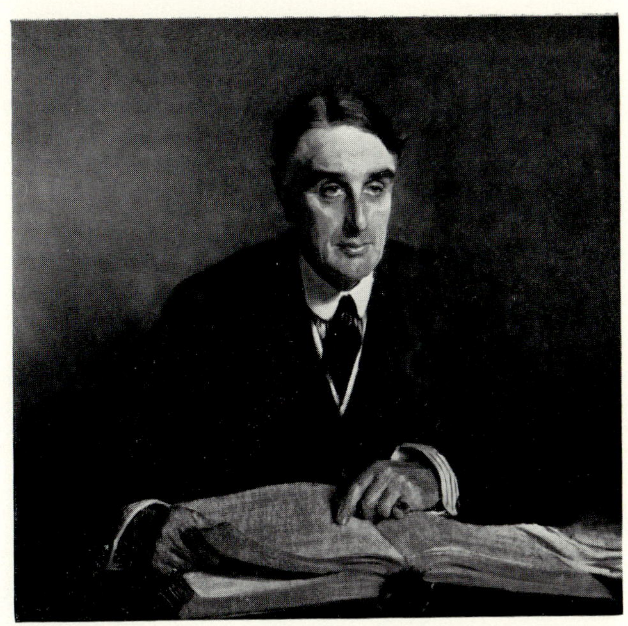

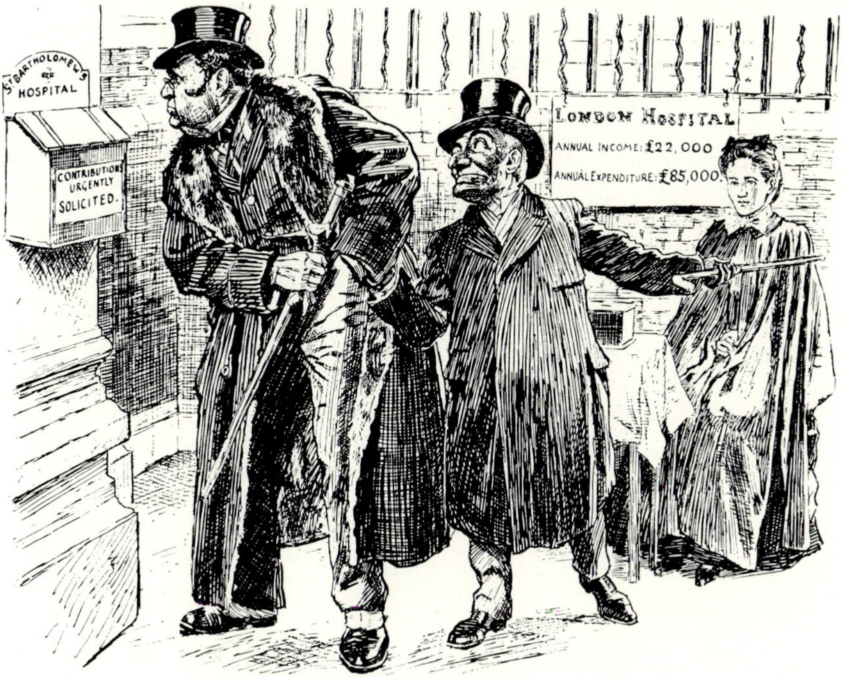

THE GREATER NEED
Sydney Holland, caricatured as Punch
(*Reproduced by permission of Punch*)

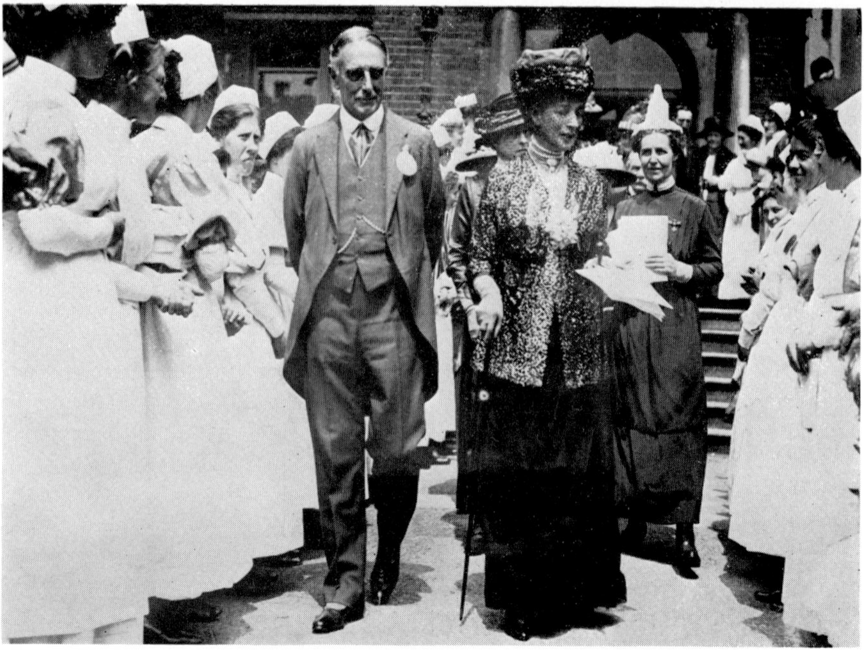

QUEEN ALEXANDRA VISITING THE HOSPITAL

FINSEN LIGHT DEPARTMENT

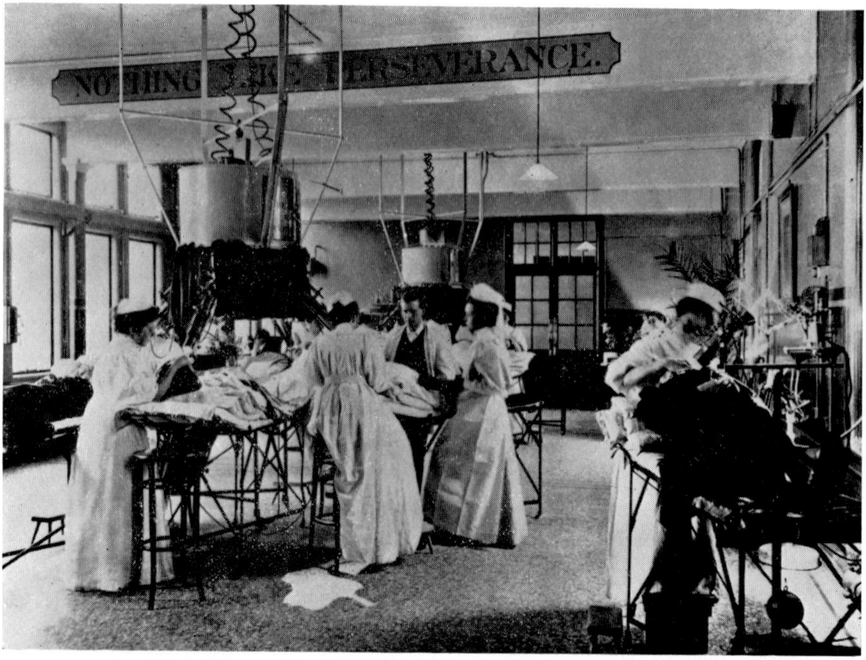

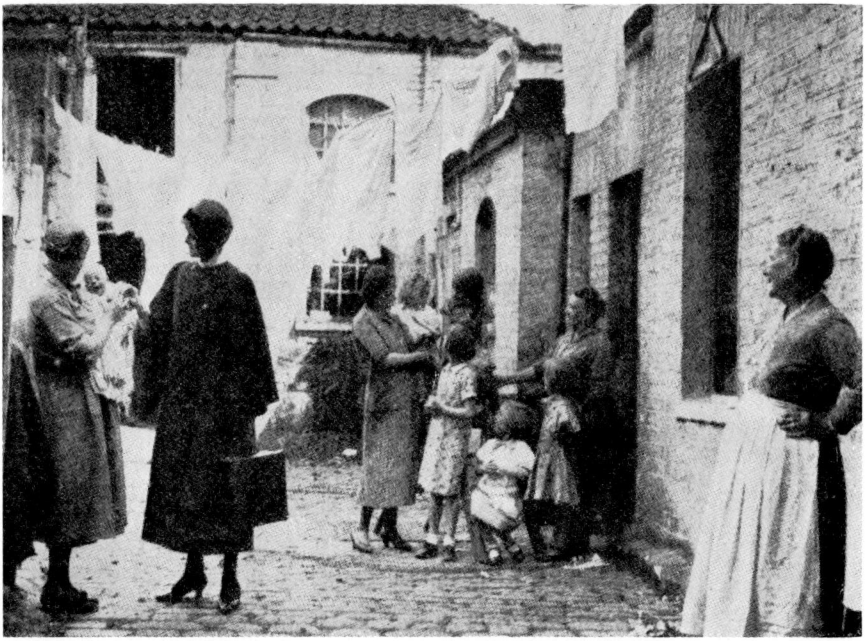

THE 'GREEN' MATERNITY CHARITY

MARIE CELESTE PATIENTS IN 1915

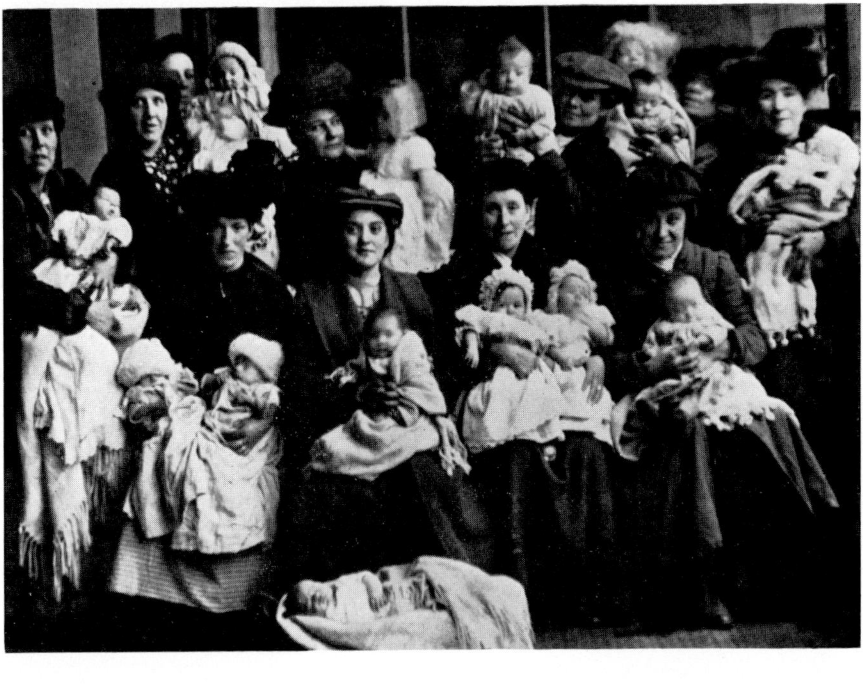

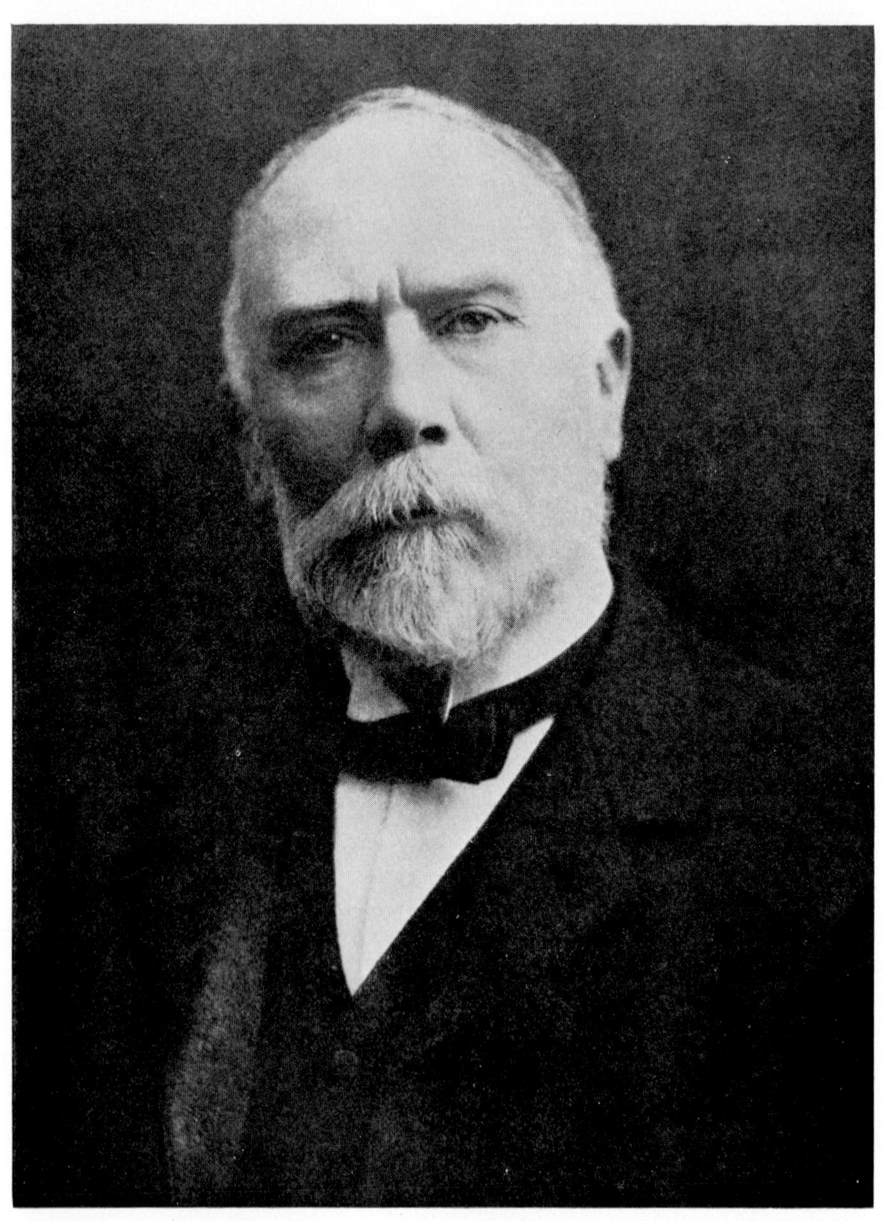

SIR JAMES MACKENZIE, F.R.S.

governors in the library of the medical college, the only room big enough to hold the large number expected to attend. The chairman opened the proceedings and, in moving the adoption of the report of the house committee, said that the Lords had gone out of their way to inquire in detail into nursing at 'the London' simply because certain former probationers had offered themselves as witnesses of their own accord. He had complete confidence in the matron. This was too much for Mrs Hunter. She rose immediately and proposed an amendment to the report, deprecating any confidence whatever on the part of the governors in her. This was quickly, heavily and vociferously defeated, but a special sub-committee was appointed to consider and report on the various allegations that had been made against the hospital in the Lords.

It had been said, this committee reported in due course, that too much power in the hospital was vested in the matron. On the contrary, they found that the hospital was run on the lines laid down as desirable by Miss Nightingale, and that the matron's power did not differ from that of the matrons of most other hospitals. It had been said that untrained nurses had been sent out to nurse private patients. This was not so. At most hospitals one year was regarded as adequate for training and, although at 'the London' a certificate was not granted until the end of two, no probationer with under one year's training had ever been sent out to nurse a private case. Neither was it true that the food was bad or that too much menial work was required of their nurses. Nor did too much responsibility rest on the shoulders of untrained nurses. An inexperienced probationer had never been left in sole charge of a serious case and, when a ward was heavy, the proportion of one sister, two staff nurses and two probationers by day, and one staff nurse and two probationers by night, to every thirty patients, had always been maintained. The report concluded: 'Whatever the work may be, the duties of the nursing staff are discharged with a self-devotion which deserves the highest praise. We are asked, it appears, to institute against our Matron a searching public enquiry. We cannot conceive any course which would be more unjust.'

When this report was debated at the next meeting of the governors, again in the library of the medical college, Mrs Hunter, speaking 'amid growing manifestations of impatience', appealed to her fellow governors not to rely on their committee but to go into these matters for themselves. This was too much for Sir Hay Currie. He rose and indignantly condemned the unfounded attacks that had been made on the management of the hospital. The injury inflicted on it by them had been incalculable, he said. 'There was no overwork; no underfeeding (cheers). It was simply a case of one woman getting her knife into another woman. (Prolonged cheers.)' This in turn was too much for Mrs Hunter, who rose again to declare (amid noisy protests) that, until the Select Committee sat, she had known nothing about the matron. Mr Yatman then spoke and, in spite of being repeatedly interrupted by cries of 'sit down' and 'divide', proposed an amendment to the effect that 'active steps should be taken to improve the nursing at "the London" during the coming year'. This was seconded by Mr Hall, most of whose speech was drowned by noisy protests. On a show of hands Mr Yatman's amendment was then rejected by 150 votes to 4, and the report of the sub-committee adopted.

This debate was reported in the public press, and Mrs Bedford Fenwick's *Nursing Record* published a long supplement condemning the denial of the right of free speech at the last meeting of the court of governors of the London Hospital. The *Pall Mall Gazette* also returned to the attack. 'So long as nursing at "the London" is mainly performed by learners, so long as women are worked eighty-four hours in the week, so long as girls just entering upon the trying ordeal of hospital life are only allowed a week's holiday at the end of each six months, so long as probationers are sent out as trained nurses, so long nursing arrangements at the hospital will continue to excite unfavourable comments.' This was too much even for the nurses themselves. Goaded into action, they wrote to the house committee. 'We object,' they said, 'being represented as a down-trodden spineless body of weak, incapable discontented women, thinking of nothing but our food and our off-duty times, and regarding it as a trouble to attend to the wants of the patients and unable to fight our own battles, if need be.'

The Lords, having devoted ten whole sessions to 'the London', got through all the rest of the metropolitan hospitals, both voluntary and poor law, in thirty, making it look more than ever as if a dead set had been made at 'the London'. But it was not until June 1892, by which time most of the excitement had died down, that their report was published. The hospitals, they found, were well administered. They had been impressed by the work of the unpaid governors of the voluntary ones but commented unfavourably on their uneven distribution in relation to the poorer districts. East and south-east London were particularly short of beds. The medical schools, they said, could properly affiliate themselves to the University, and thereby acquire first-rate teachers in the pre-clinical subjects, and they deplored the fact that the poor-law infirmaries were not used for clinical teaching. In regard to nurses' working hours and holidays, they were, in relation to the condition of most of the hospitals at this date, probably unrealistic, and certainly idealistic when they came down in favour of Mrs Bedford Fenwick's contention that it took three years to train a nurse. (Miss Nightingale still thought one enough; Miss Lückes two.) The charges against 'the London', they said, had been made mainly by persons who had grievances of their own. These had not been substantiated by other evidence, and had been adequately refuted by the matron and the medical staff. The nurse–patient ratio there was no lower, and the work of the nurses no harder, than at most other hospitals. 'In justice to "the London" the Committee wish to add that it is an admirable hospital doing excellent work in a part of London where it confers innumerable benefits upon a very large and very poor population.'

The attacks on 'the London', it seems certain, were largely prompted by personal animosity. No other hospital was attacked in respect of its nursing in the same venomous way before the Select Committee of the Lords, but in all probability there was some substance in the accusations levelled against it which all those loyal to it naturally wanted to cover up. 'The London' had outgrown itself. There is no doubt about that. With inadequate funds it was attempting an impossible task, the matron being faced with the insoluble problem of nursing too many patients with too few nurses, simply due to lack of accommodation for them. Inevitably they were overworked; their hours on duty too long; their time off too short. The truth is, that under the inspired leadership of a matron who believed passionately in the need for all-out dedication to nursing, the hospital had been running on women who were prepared to overwork and risk their health in the service of the sick. The small minority, unprepared to sacrifice themselves in this way, and jealous of those who did, had caused most of the trouble.

Gradually the talk of scandals at 'the London' died down, and the nursing at it ceased to be news value, but not before incalculable damage had been done. The hospital had been heavily criticized in public and then forced to wait a whole year to be vindicated. Mud slung tends to stick, too, whatever amends are made later, and the Select Committee of the Lords had wrecked the prestige of 'the London' in the eyes of the general public. Subscriptions had fallen off and it soon stood thousands of pounds in debt although the demands on its services remained just as great as ever. 'The pressure on the beds remains very heavy', wrote the house committee in their report in 1896. 'There is an average of well over 700 patients in the Hospital, and when the wards are so full all the cases are of an exceptionally severe character; and the strain on the staff proportionally great. Again and again extra beds have to be put up to avoid sending patients away. Numerous cases of scarlet fever and diphtheria are brought to "the London", the majority of which are simply removed to their own home by the Metropolitan Asylums Board who have no accommodation for the treatment of these cases, and again we are forced to take in the severe ones in spite of our facilities for isolating being utterly inadequate.' 'The London' was also falling back in the quality of its service to the public; failing to keep up to date in the face of the demands created by recent advances in medical science and technology. In spite of anaesthetics and the modern antiseptic techniques, there was still only one operating theatre. In spite of Röntgen's discovery, there was still only a shed in the garden for

X-ray work. In spite of increasing knowledge in bacteriology, there was still no clinical laboratory. There was no proper out-patient department, no adequate facilities for isolation, no electric power. The wards were in urgent need of renovation, the whole building far too small.

Pessimism prevailed. Nothing could be done without money, and where was that coming from now? The chairman of that date, although hard-working, lacked knowledge, vision and drive. The house committee were elderly, timid and unimaginative, and many governors wondering, from what they were told, how long the charity would be able to carry on at all. They did not know, and how could they have known, that the man to match the hour was at hand?

12

Prince of Beggars

In 1896 Sydney Holland, later second Viscount Knutsford (and it is Knutsford that I shall call him, for it is as Knutsford that those left who knew him remember him), was just forty and had already been Chairman of Poplar Hospital for some time. His connection with the East End had been accidental. Under his uncle's will, he had become a shareholder in the East and West India Dock Company, and in the 'tanner a day' dock strike round about this date, he had gone out of his way to state what he believed to be the legitimate grievances of the men. He had also begun to take an interest in their welfare, and the conditions under which they worked; hence frequent visits to Poplar Hospital, where he had soon become a governor. Then he had been elected chairman and proceeded to transform it from a pokey little place with thirty beds into a modern hospital with over a hundred. By besieging the public, too, he had raised its reserve funds from eight to over fifty thousand pounds.

So, as the chairmanship of 'the London' now seemed likely to fall vacant, several governors, it would appear, asked him to join them and stand at the next elections for the house committee. 'I did not know Miss Lückes, but I knew her by reputation', he was to write many years later, 'so I called on her, and she advised me to stand, and in a way I can never forget, pointed out the possibilities, if one would devote one's life to hospital work and not make it just one of many occupations. She told me of her own aims and ambitions and ideals for nurses and of her difficulties, and ended,

"I suppose you would not come here? I would serve you loyally. We are in need of energetic help."'

So Knutsford was elected to the house committee of 'the London' and set to work to grasp the complexities of that vast institution. He was appalled by what he found.

'There was a blight over everything', he wrote. 'No one seemed to have visioned the great forward movement in hospital administration that was hurrying to its birth. There was only one operating theatre and only one table, a wooden affair like those in butchers' shops. Aseptic surgery was just coming in but the staff were still doubtful about it. When a surgeon went round he was followed by the beadle who carried a baize-covered tray containing instruments which were used and re-used with complete disregard of the principles of asepsis. One tiny room sufficed for bacteriological work; a shed in the garden was all the accommodation "the London" could spare for X-ray work. Most of the nurses lived a "Box and Cox life" and many in the small houses in the district. There was only one Home. On the financial side the position was depressing. The subscriptions for 1895 had fallen to only £8750. The public had lost interest and possessed even less faith in the Hospital. Nevertheless, what I saw impressed me with the ambition to put things right. So I set to work, and worked as I had never worked before in all my life.'

By the end of the year he had his report ready on all that was needed to be done to bring 'the London' up to date, in his own words, up to 'what the largest hospital in England ought to be'. The arrangements for dealing with out-patients were utterly inadequate. The waiting-hall was in the basement corridor and patients seen in little rooms opening out of it. A completely new department above ground was needed; special wards for osteomyelitis, puerperal septicaemia and other septic diseases, all common in those days; an isolation block for cases of the acute infectious fevers brought up too ill to be transferred to fever hospitals. The bacteriological cause of many diseases had now been discovered, so a bacteriological laboratory was needed. Röntgen's recent discovery was bound to be exploited in the service of medicine, so more space would soon be required for an X-ray department. There were nine surgeons on the staff, but still only one operating theatre; over 650 beds, but, as they were usually occupied by accidents and acute cases, the waiting lists for semi-urgent cases were growing longer and longer. Special wards for children, ophthalmic wards, observation wards and wards for mental cases were also required. More beds had to be provided somehow. Balconies were wanted so that patients could be wheeled out into the sunshine, the fresh air treatment for tuber-culosis being attempted even in Whitechapel.

Knutsford therefore startled the governors by suggesting in his report, not only that the whole hospital, now in a shocking state of disrepair both internally and externally, should be renovated and modernized, but also that its walls should be reinforced and Mainwaring's old building pushed up two storeys higher! The necessity for doing this and for carrying out his many other recommendations was unassailable. But who was to raise the money for doing it and, if it could be raised, who was to carry them out? There was clearly only one answer to that; the author of the 'bomb-shell report', as it came to be called, himself. Would he be prepared to devote the same amount of energy to 'the London', he was asked, as he had already devoted to Poplar? His answer was that he would. So the chairman resigned, and in December 1896 Knutsford was elected in his place.

On two major questions of policy he immediately joined issue with the house committee. Out-patients, he said, who could afford to pay something should contribute towards the cost of the medicines and bandages with which they were provided. This was reluctantly conceded. More controversial still was his revolu-tionary proposal that governors' letters should be abolished. The large majority of patients in the house, it is true, were accidents or acute medical cases; in respect of them 'the London' was already a 'free' hospital. To all others, the old system of governors' letters still, theoretically at least, applied; governors were still entitled to recommend sixteen patients a year and patients sent up with these letters were always admitted, if the severity of their illness demanded it and there was a bed available. This sounds fair enough. But there was good reason to suppose, he had found, that many of these were often admitted over the heads of more deserving patients. In short, as we would say today, they 'jumped the queue'. Knutsford now argued that admissions must be based, not on whether a patient had a letter from a governor or not, but entirely on his or her degree of poverty and medical condition. Admission by governor's letter was, however, a vested interest. The new chairman soon deemed it politic to withdraw his proposal for the time being.

Nothing could be done without money, and Knutsford, in stating the conditions under which he would accept the chairmanship, had insisted that all appeal work should rest solely in his own hands. The house committee had been only too ready to agree, and he now began his great campaign to raise money for the charity. He sat down to write, in article after article, and stood up to talk, in speech after speech, on its behalf. He mobilized the pulpit and the press. He raised money out of laughter and conjured up cheques out of tears. He wrote letter after letter, many of these thousands a personal duel with a chosen antagonist, again and again a deliberate attempt to get past the guard of indifference or preoccupation which his adversary put up, and reach his heart. Sometimes he played on the sentimental string; at others he relied on hard facts – and he had plenty of them ready – tellingly set out. Often he took risks. Again and again, when he thought a cheque too small, he would tear it up and send back the bits, demanding more. And often got it!

In the very first year of his chairmanship he scored a big success. He wrote to Alfred Yarrow, the shipping magnate, explaining his urgent need for a new out-patient building. In reply he received £3000. Knutsford did not think this from a man like that anything like enough. 'Come and see the Hospital', he wrote back. Yarrow came and saw and Knutsford conquered. 'I'll give you £25000 to remedy this,' said Yarrow, 'provided my name is kept out of it', and at the same time asked whether Knutsford would like any special conditions attached to the gift? Knutsford took a risk. 'Make it conditional on the abolition of governors' letters!' and the house committee, afraid to look a gift horse in the mouth, capitulated.

Shortly after this Edward Raphael gave £10000 to endow the Jewish wards. Then Knutsford got a message from a Mr Fielden asking him to call. 'I went round and found quite a young man', writes Knutsford. 'He had recently been operated on by Sir Frederick Treves, who had told him that I wanted help for the London Hospital, and now asked me to write down what I wanted. I started with £100 for something and went up to a complete isolation block costing £22000.' Fielden immediately wrote him a cheque for that amount. In the same year, too, James Hora, beset with the fear that he had neglected his wife, expressed a wish to endow some part of the hospital which could bear her name. Knutsford suggested the Samaritan Society to which Hora now covenanted a large annual subscription. So it now became the Marie Celeste Samaritan Society. Mr Hora also endowed the Marie Celeste maternity wards and left £120000 to the Samaritan Society in his will. This was typical of Knutsford's way of doing things, but it does seem a pity that the Samaritan Society, founded by Blizard in the eighteenth century and the first society of its kind, should have become associated with an obscure nineteenth-century lady who had never had any connection with the hospital.

In 1898 Knutsford was taking Mr B. W. Levy round the hospital when they came across a group of men sitting draped in those red blankets which were such a familiar feature of the wards until the second war. He asked who they were. They were waiting for operation, he was told, but, as there was only one theatre, some of them might drop off the end of the queue that day in the sense that their operations would have to be postponed. Mr Levy: 'Do you really tell me that you put a man to all this anxiety and waiting, and then you do not operate after all?' Knutsford had to admit that it could happen. It was the inevitable consequence of only having one theatre. 'This cannot be allowed to go on', exclaimed Levy. 'Give me a piece of paper.' And he wrote Knutsford a cheque for £13000, adding, 'I give you this on condition that these new theatres are open to all men of all creeds [he was a strict Jew] for all time, and that my name is never mentioned in connection with them as long as I am still alive.'

In the same year as Mr Levy's benefaction the quinquennial appeal – the voluntary hospitals had agreed among themselves to arrange their appeals so that they did not clash – raised £55000, but much more was needed if Knutsford's bomb-shell report was to be fully implemented. So he now approached the Prince of Wales Hospital Fund (later King Edward VII Fund) for London, – which had been set up to help all the voluntary hospitals – and this body, having inspected the hospital and studied his reconstruction plans, promised an annual grant of £5000, on condition that the hospital, on its part, spent £100000 of capital in putting them into effect. By the turn of the century the reconstruction of the hospital, according to Knutsford's plans, was already in full swing.

War had now broken out in South Africa, and our soldiers had gone out to fight in the same scarlet uniforms as those worn in the Crimea and at Waterloo. Military disaster followed, but before long typhoid was taking a greater toll of life than all the guns and rifles of the enemy. Nursing arrangements broke down and Princess Alexandra, who had already often visited the hospital both officially and unofficially, asked Knutsford to find twenty-six nurses to go out to the war under the title of 'Princess of Wales' Nurses'. She came down to the hospital herself and gave each one a present. Treves and Openshaw, the latter an orthopaedic surgeon, went with them, and the whole party was given a great send-off at Waterloo. Treves became attached to Buller's army in Natal and served at Colenso and in the relief of Ladysmith. Nurse Clara Evans never came back. She died of typhoid in South Africa.

Soon after this Knutsford was invited down to Sandringham. This was the first of many subsequent visits of its kind. His personality appealed to the Prince, so soon to become king, and the Princess began to take more and more interest in 'the London'. 'Remember that the London Hospital is *my* hospital', she said to him one day, 'and I wish to be President of it.' So, when Queen Victoria died in January 1901 and in June of the following year, the King, now all set for his coronation, was suddenly taken ill at Sandringham with what we now know to be acute appendicitis –

a condition then only vaguely recognized – what was more natural than that Treves, now the leading abdominal surgeon in London, should be called in consultation? The King refused operation and, a week later, insisted on travelling to London for his coronation. That night he did not feel so well and Lord Lister, Sir Thomas Barlow and Sir Frederick Treves were called in consultation. All agreed that operation was imperative. Again the King refused: he would not disappoint the nation. He was determined to go to the Abbey. 'Then, Sir, you will go there as a dead man', Treves is said to have told him.

Reluctantly the King consented and Treves telegraphed Knutsford. Would he send a nurse to the Palace at once? The King was very ill and he would be operating on him next day. Sir Stanley Hewitt (also on the staff of 'the London') would give the anaesthetic. 'The Queen told me afterwards', wrote Knutsford, 'that the King walked into the operating room, improvised by Nurse Haines, in his oldest dressing gown, of which she felt quite ashamed, and climbed up on the table without help. She stayed on in the room until he was insensible.'

Fielden's isolation block had come into action in the year that Queen Victoria died. Mr Levy's theatres were opened in the year of the operation on the King, and in the following summer the King himself, whose life in the eyes of the public, had been saved by a London Hospital surgeon, opened the new out-patient building. An inconspicuous figure in the back row on the platform was Alfred Yarrow, whose munificent gift had alone rendered its construction possible.

Meanwhile, the whole hospital was rising by two storeys, and the confusion was indescribable. But there was no confusion of purpose. The chairman, with his sense of humour, his passion for sport, his approachability, his capacity for making friends, and above all his deep and genuine sense of pity, about which there is no doubt, had caught the imagination and inspired the enthusiasm of staff and students, of nurses and lay workers, of scrubbers and cleaners, in fact of all and sundry. Raising money for so good a cause had become the same exciting game for all. Of course he enjoyed it. And why not? He would make 'the London' the largest, and make it the best, hospital in the country. It was the heyday of the voluntary system. Politics and class feeling had not yet spoilt the spirit of service which inspired it.

He had now shown himself to be as able at organization as he was good at raising money, and soon saw that the administration of the hospital was over-centralized. Every department was now put under an executive officer, responsible to a sub-committee of the house committee, and whose relationship to the chairman of this sub-committee corresponded to that of the permanent secretary of a government department to his political chief. In addition to nursing, household management and catering, there were now theatre floor, out-patient, accounts, and surveyors' departments. (Only the appeal department remained directly under Knutsford.) So the house governor's job had changed. He was no longer top-dog administrator. Rather, his was the more difficult task of integrating the decisions of these committees and supervising the work of their executive officers. Knutsford's quick judgement of character had here stood him in good stead. He had chosen E. W. Morris as chief dispenser, and he had saved the hospital £1000 in his first year of office. So, when the new theatre floor came into action, Morris was asked to take it over. 'After a week spent seeing how things were done at other hospitals, and a second at a surgical instrument makers, Morris organized the department so admirably that it has worked without a hitch ever since.' When the more than ever important post of house governor became vacant, Morris was appointed to it. 'The organization of the hospital today', Knutsford was to write in 1926, 'stands as the monument to his success.'

In 1904 the Duke of Cambridge died. He had been president for over half a century. There was no doubt as to who his successor would be. 'The London Hospital is *my* hospital', Queen Alexandra had said, 'and I wish to be President of it', and it was through its new president that 'the London' now became the first hospital in Britain to start the treatment of lupus (tuberculous disease of the skin) by means of Finsen's mercury vapour lamp. For Queen Alexandra was a Dane, and it was natural that she wished to see the treatment for it, started by Finsen in her own country, adopted in what had now become her own hospital. The medical profession was sceptical. So was Knutsford from what he had heard, but she persuaded him to send Sir Stephen Mackenzie, on whom Andrew Clark's mantle of wise physician had now fallen, and two nurses, to Copenhagen to study Finsen's methods. They returned convinced. 'The start [of our light department]', writes Knutsford, 'was appalling. From all parts of England and from every corner of the globe miserable beings who had hidden themselves away from the sight of their fellows (the disease starts on and destroys the face) hurried to "the London". In a few days we had a waiting list for two whole years ahead.'

By 1906 the reconstruction of the hospital was virtually complete. For five years it had been in the hands of the builders and renovators; not a single ward exempt. The difficulty of carrying on its work with gangs of workmen wandering about and constructional operations in progress almost everywhere must have been immense. Corridors had been repeatedly blocked, necessitating a journey to another floor and back in order to get to the other end of the same one. Lifts had been out of action; night shifts had often been necessary to get some important job done quickly. Screws had been used instead of nails to put down floors, merely to save noise, and at much increased expense. On one occasion all work in the east wing had been suspended for a whole day for the sake of one patient for whom sleep was held essential. And yet, when the temporary ward put up in the garden had been pulled down, the builders had cleared up their mess, and the last workman had stolen silently away, the routine work of the hospital had never been seriously interrupted. Never had a ward been closed or a single bed put out of action.

This orgy of building and reconstruction, including building a new nurses' home in Oxford Street (now Stepney Way), had cost the then enormous sum of £450000. Knutsford had suffered many anxious moments. Would he ever succeed in raising the money to pay for the vast scheme to which he had committed the hospital? 'In 1903 we were in great despair,' he writes, 'and as I was passing the Mansion House one day, an inspiration seized me to go in and see the Lord Mayor and ask him if he would help.' Lord Bearsted did help. He gave a Mansion House dinner in aid of the charity entirely at his own expense, the first of its kind ever held, and this raised a lot of money. In the same anxious year, too, a special appeal launched by Bart's threatened to undercut 'the London's' legitimate quinquennial, but right was on Knutsford's side and he succeeded in getting round the editor of *Punch* who published a cartoon, caricaturing him as Punch pointing to a London and away from a Bart's nurse. 'Excuse me, Mr Bull, but this is where the money is most needed.' So the quinquennial appeal that year proved the most successful in the whole history of the hospital. It raised £134000.

The hospital had had to sell out £100000 of stock and raise £40000 out of the sale of land, so the income of the charity had been alarmingly reduced while the cost of running it had increased enormously. It now maintained 900 beds with an average of over 800 patients in the house at any one time; over 14000 in-patients and over 200000 out-patients were now under treatment every year. Knutsford continued to be anxious: it was a hand-to-mouth existence. But subscriptions, legacies and appeals continued to make ends meet.

He chose the executive officer and the chairman of each departmental sub-committee himself. They reported directly to him, and in this way the work of the house committee was kept down to policy, and time spent talking was cut to the bone. Never did he allow a fixed agenda; that, in his opinion, merely led to useless talk. He decided what the committee ought to decide in advance and then, in the fewest possible words, got them to decide it for themselves. His increasing deafness sometimes proved an embarrassment to him, but far more often he used it as an ally on his side. Some controversial items on his unpublished agenda would have been settled before he 'heard' the criticism levelled at it. Or, bored by some long-winded speaker, he would switch off his enormous box-like hearing aid ostentatiously. Then everyone tittered and the troublesome gentleman sat down. Further, again and again he would call on his irrepressible sense of humour and fund of good stories, often against himself, to help him out on a sticky wicket. His handling of the house committee has been described as farcical and the court of governors could always be relied upon to sign on the dotted line. He was indeed an autocratic chairman. But he was the kind of dictator who makes few mistakes. He had also gathered round him men both anxious and competent to help him.

His, too, was the personal touch. He lunched at the hospital every day. He knew everybody; doctors, nurses, porters, cleaners; and not only them themselves but their lives, their circumstances and their troubles, too. He visited every department repeatedly. He delighted in going round the wards and talking to the nurses and patients. He entertained the children, and adults, too, with his amateur conjuring. How well even I remember him – many years later than this, of course – entertaining a boy in my ward, who was to have an egg for his tea, by making it disappear and then reappear from behind his own head. Unfortunately, it had not yet been boiled and the worst occurred. I can see him now, standing ruefully in his habitual morning coat and striped trousers, being wiped down by sister in the lobby.

He regarded the medical staff with caution and, because he saw danger in allowing them too much say in matters of administration and policy, was vigilant in preserving the over-riding power of the governors and their lay committee. Nor was he interested in science as such. It had barely begun to grow into education yet. Medicine interested him only as a means to an end: getting ill people well. Patients came first, and all other interests must always be subordinated to theirs. With this end in view he strove to meet the requirements of the medical staff as far as he could, but he kept his eye on them. If an operation had not been performed after a patient had been prepared for it, Knutsford must know the reason why, and, if there was no sufficient reason, he struck and struck hard. On one occasion, it is said, he forced the resignation of a surgeon who had left a patient on his list at the hospital to operate on a private one in the West End. Occasionally, too, his perceptive judgement of character led him to differ from that of the medical staff, and there are instances of young men of unproved ability whose feet were set on the ladder of success by Knutsford's choice against the verdict of the profession.

In spite of this, he got on with the doctors. 'I wonder', he wrote, 'if any hospital chairman has ever had happier relations with his staff. We have disagreed, we have fought, and we have stayed friends.'

F

13

Great Partnership

'After long years of struggle alone,' Miss Lückes had written to Miss Nightingale in 1896, 'I have found a helper who is genuinely interested and believes in the importance of all and everything that we are trying to do.' For just as Knutsford had become interested in the lives of the dockers in Poplar, so on election to the chairmanship, realizing the importance of good nursing, he had taken a special interest in the work and lives of the nurses and become champion of their cause. 'It was Miss Lückes who asked me to come to the Hospital,' he was to write years later, 'and since then I have seen her or written to her, not occasionally, but literally every day, and I have telephoned her almost every night.'

Nursing at a large hospital at that date was in many ways very different to what it is now. Apart from vaccination, preventive innoculation had hardly yet begun and many diseases were common then which are rarely seen today. Nor was there yet any effective way of treating most of them; no chemotherapy for septic infection, tuberculosis or pneumonia; no insulin for diabetes (all young diabetics died); no liver extract or vitamin B2 for pernicious anaemia; no radiotherapy for malignant growth. Treatment was still in the main symptomatic. Surgery, too, although often successful, was heavily handicapped by blood transfusion not being practicable as yet, and the serious risks of open anaesthesia. So the mortality of all diseases was much higher than it is today, and the expectation of life of all ages correspondingly lower. Relatively few lived to get cancer or to suffer strokes. They died too young.

Infants were admitted with laryngeal obstruction, necessitating immediate tracheotomy, though still many died. 'I was on duty all Sunday in charge of a special ward for children with dip,' wrote a probationer in 1906, 'dashing from cot to cot, in case babies coughed out their tracheotomy tube. Many tracheotomies were done, particularly at week-ends, on Jewish children because their parents would not bring them up until after midnight on Saturday.'

Epidemic diarrhoea and vomiting in infants (*cholera infantum*) was still rife with its frightful mortality, largely due to the ignorance still prevailing as to the mechanism of water–salt balance in the body and consequent lack of knowledge as to how to handle dehydration. 'A depressing time,' writes the same probationer, 'babies dying like flies due to a bad epidemic of D and V; children quite emaciated when admitted. Night Staff (nurse) coping with those she hopes will live, while nurse W. and I sit all night making shrouds and laying out these mites. Fourteen died.' Every children's ward, too, would contain its quota of rheumatic fever (rarely seen now), with its swollen painful joints, and cases of St Vitus' dance, the uncontrolled movements associated with it often so violent that precautions had to be taken to stop children throwing themselves out of bed. Both predisposed the patient to valvular disease of the heart, leading to failure and death from it in early adult life.

Puerperal septicaemia was common and could devastate a ward (there was no penicillin then to treat it with). In local infection, inflammation was still encouraged by the application of heat and 'laudable' pus let out as soon as it had formed. Multiple incisions were often necessary. In acute osteomyelitis and mastoid-itis dead bone had to be removed with mallet and chisel, and the resulting cavity packed with gauze, necessitating repeated and often painful dressings.

Respiratory infection dominated the nursing in all medical, and complicated it in many surgical, wards. Broncho-pneumonia was a common cause of death, both in infants and the elderly; it was the cause of the high death rate in the epidemic of influenza which swept the country in 1889. It was a common complication then of all operations under general anaesthesia. It was almost inevitable, too, in any elderly patient compelled to take to bed for any great length of time. Many who had fractured their femur died of it. Lobar pneumonia, which seems to have almost disappeared now, was also common then, coming 'out of the blue', at least so it seemed, and striking down many a hefty working man. Twenty per cent died. The rest recovered completely.

Typhoid and typhus were still endemic and nursed in general wards. Tuberculosis was common. In children it took the form of meningitis, invariably fatal, or of chronic inflammation of glands, bones and joints. In adults infection of the lungs was the rule, leading to coughing, progressive loss of weight and spitting blood. Most consumptives, as the disease was then called, faded out in the infirmaries, but it would sometimes flare up suddenly into the 'galloping consumption', dramatized so often by playwrights to provide the death of their heroine on the stage. These cases were admitted to the general hospitals.

Acute abdominal conditions, such as acute appendicitis, strangulated hernia, perforated gastric and duodenal ulcer seem to have been much more common then. At least, one is left with that impression. In consequence there were many more urgent abdominal operations and the post-operative nursing of them was often heavy. On the other hand, there was much less 'cold' surgery. Anaesthesia at that date with all its attendant risks did not permit the many things and lengthy operations the surgeons safely do today. The surgery of the brain, chest and heart had hardly yet begun.

The outcome of an illness, particularly of a medical illness, would again and again depend largely on good nursing; on the hot-packs and poultices to promote inflammation; on the tepid sponging to keep down fever; on the careful lifting to counter pain and trauma; on the repeated turning to prevent bed sores; on the invalid cooking and persuasive feeding to maintain nutrition. Whether a particular patient survived pneumonia or typhoid, for instance, often turned, not so much on anything particular that the doctor did, but on the efficiency with which the nurses exercised their art.

So the nurse–patient relationship mattered far more, in a kind of way, than it does today. The nurses' twelve-hour day, with alternate night and day shifts, and minimum time off compatible with enough sleep and maintenance of physical health, was tacitly accepted. Nothing else was taken into serious account. Continuity was essential to good nursing (the eight-hour day would have been something inconceivable then). When a patient was critically ill, as in lobar pneumonia with the patient heading for the crisis, the sister would stay on duty as long as she could before handing over to the night staff, in order to see him through it. No one saw anything out of the ordinary in that then.

The attitude which nurses were expected to adopt to their work was also rather different. In the first place, the emancipation of women was not yet a reality. No woman of the upper or middle class expected the kind of life that women in them live today. In the second, as Miss Lückes had told the Select Committee of the Lords, a nurse was 'not an ordinary woman or she would not have taken up nursing as a profession'. A hospital nurse was, or should be, of the kind prepared to dedicate her life to her work, and no more look for emotional satisfaction outside it than a nun in a convent should look for it outside the love of God. To Miss Lückes nursing had always been, and to Knutsford nursing was now soon to become, the most exalted profession that any woman – although neither of them was particularly religious – could adopt, demanding as it did maximum service and personal sacrifice. Marriage and nursing meant divided loyalty and were generally regarded as incompatible. A woman who wanted to marry must give up nursing or at least hospital nursing; so the nurses then were unmarried, and most of the sisters middle aged, although women of character and with vast experience of the seamy side of life. This view, held at all the voluntary hospitals – 'the London' possessed no monopoly of it – may seem absurd to us now, but it was the philosophy of Miss Nightingale and the pioneers. It was the foundation on which the spirit of British nursing was built in the late nineteenth century.

Dedication to their work was certainly required of all nurses at 'the London'. When Knutsford took over as chairman, he had found the matron struggling to nurse an average of 800 patients, most of them serious accidents and cases of acute illness and over a thousand dying in the hospital every year, with only 230 nurses. She had no sleeping accommodation for more. It was an impossible situation, hard, in fact, to believe that she could cope with it at all. Knutsford was appalled. 'You must come and tell the house committee all that you want to put nursing at the London on its feet.' At least another hundred nurses, she had told them, and another hundred beds to sleep them in. This, she had said, would give her 36 more nurses by day and another 24 by night, and ensure a reserve of about 40 to provide against sickness and holidays. So a new nurses' home had been included in Knutsford's plans as a high priority. This was now building south of Oxford Street, or Stepney Way as it has since been re-named.

Until that was ready Knutsford and Miss Lückes strove to ease the burden the nurses carried without reducing their standard of service to their patients. This was managed in a number of small ways. The broken-down old bedsteads, mostly very low and of all shapes and sizes, many still of wood, too, had been an eyesore in the hospital for years. High ones, all of metal and improved pattern, now took their place in all the wards. This lightened the nurses' work, with all the heavy lifting it entailed. New lockers and bed tables to fit the beds were also provided. Mr Cotes, a governor, started a fund in his newspaper, *The Sun*, to raise money to buy feather pillows for all the beds, to take the place of the old flock-filled ones. On the last Christmas Day of the nineteenth century all heads in the hospital rested on a pillow of this kind. In order to save the nurses climbing stairs, a bridge was constructed between the old nurses' home and the new Alexandra home. A sick room was provided on the ground floor of the latter; no longer were nurses to be admitted to the general wards when they were taken ill.

On 16 October 1906 the new nurses' home was opened at long last, but not by royalty as the Alexandra home had been. By special request of the house committee, it was opened by Miss Lückes and called 'the Lückes home' after her. This was an honour richly deserved. She had already served the hospital for twenty-five years, in fact spent half her life in it already. She had seen it through hard times. She had faced the Lords and, after standing up to so much unjust criticism, had put nursing at 'the London' on its feet. 'One hundred nurses moved over that day,' she wrote of this great occasion, 'amidst much excitement, and the three following ones were occupied with gathering together all those who had been located in temporary quarters while awaiting this longed-for event. We now have 432 bedrooms for nurses exclusive of 82 for Sisters.' More staff could now be engaged and more time off allowed. Three months later the chairman announced that it would now be possible to give the entire nursing staff one month's holiday in every year.

Her nurses still worked fantastically hard, however, according to modern standards, although probably no harder than at any other hospital at this date. The day staff came on at 7 a.m. and went off at 9.20 p.m., during which they were allowed three hours off duty and one whole day off every month. The latter they forfeited if they were late coming on duty more than six times. All classes and lectures still had to be attended in off-duty times and were organized accordingly. The night nurses came on at 9 p.m., when they could be seen hurrying across the garden carrying bits and pieces for their midnight supper, which they cooked in the ward. (The 'pro' was expected to make a pudding for the staff nurse.) They came off duty at 8 a.m. and then did their homework, writing up their lecture notes in the day room under sister's supervision. Then they were allowed out until 1 p.m., when they were required to go to bed. At 7 p.m. they were called to attend a lecture by a member of the staff. Many heads nodded. (In the late twenties the same system was still in force, and I gave those lectures myself.) This routine and the spirit of it were accepted as a matter of course. 'The amazing thing was,' wrote a sister of that date, 'that everyone accepted the discipline, the long hours, and the small salaries.' 'Tired, Nurse?' exclaimed Dame Alicia Lloyd Still, matron of St Thomas's

Hospital, to my sister, training there just before the First World War, 'You should glory in your tiredness!' That was the spirit still expected of all nurses.

Two years before Knutsford was elected chairman, Miss Lückes had started annual letters to her staff, keeping them informed of everything that was going on and emphasizing the difficulties with which a hospital supported entirely by voluntary contributions always had to contend. There can have been little encouraging to tell them then. But the personal touch was always there. 'I often wonder,' she wrote, 'if all of you working here have any idea of what a genuine regret it is to me to be able to see so little of you personally. All do not need special sympathy or attention at the same time, but if each one of you (when the individual need arises) will accept the repeated assurance that I am not only desirous but ready to help her at the first moment I am free to do so, she will not hesitate to give me the opportunity.' In order to establish personal contact with her staff she was also 'at home' every Tuesday evening to any member of it who cared to come (these were less formidable occasions than might have been imagined). Her nurses were also encouraged to slip notes under her front door; so, if a nurse wanted to talk to her personally, she could by-pass the ward sister under whom she happened to be working.

'Surely there can never have been a better time', she wrote in 1904, 'than the present for nurses to concentrate on renewed efforts to approach more nearly the ideal nurse which, in their best moments, all amongst us have aspired to become. This can only be attained by constant endeavour. In this our best hope lies. I have always told you that if you could once perceive the need for sympathy to be blended with technical skill, there is that within you which will enable you to rise to the occasion and to bestow services of a quality that are beyond price to those who are helpless and suffering. It is those who never willingly give less than their best who will go on finding satisfaction in their chosen work, and who will discover that from time to time their powers have increased and that they are growing richer, not only in what they receive, but in what they give. It is my desire for all nurses, and especially for all those who wear our uniform, that they will never be content with aiming at anything less satisfying than this. All will agree that the endeavour "to walk worthy of the vocation wherein we are called" is infinitely more important than professional success. Of all things let us guard against slackness, against the performance of routine duties without that true "love of the work" which sanctifies the drudgery; that love which makes the labours of the day – or of the night – worthy of our best endeavours. Nursing is an art as well as a "profession", and that very love for the work is the best incentive to become technically proficient.'

In order to get the right women to start training she interviewed every candidate herself. In Whitechapel it was peculiarly difficult to come by the right type, and in a letter to Miss Nightingale she lamented how she had to see over a thousand candidates in order to find two hundred who she seriously thought worth while taking on and into whom she hoped to be able to inculcate her high ideals. To achieve the latter she relied on her lectures, talking to the probationers in her high clear voice in a way that few nurses had ever been talked to before; not only on the technicalities of modern nursing, but on their grave responsibilities and on the ethical standards of their profession. The chairman himself listened to some of these talks, 'hidden away behind the gallery'. Before long he had been co-opted to help her. He now gave a talk to each new batch of probationers. These talks were undoubtedly impressive. He was a good talker, and in him her somewhat overpowering earnestness was corrected by his irrepressible sense of humour and his hatred of insincerity.

'I care for your happiness and for your material success', Miss Lückes wrote once, 'more than I can say. And so does Mr Holland. [He had not yet succeeded to his father's title.] We are both ready to serve you and glad of the opportunity. When we can help you, either in big things or in small, do not hesitate to ask us. In return we only want to be assured that you and your work are worthy of the reputation gained for our Hospital by many past and present Londoners with whom we are all proud to be associated. I have always particularly liked that remark in Mr Holland's talks where he asks nurses if they "cannot go up a little higher" in order to help other women to advance; and we prevent, instead of encouraging them to do this, if we pause half way up the ladder blocking the way. The danger lies in failure to recognize that this is true. The opportunities of accomplishing more are often missed, not because they do not exist, but on account of our failure to perceive them. I am impelled to say this because I see the danger of those who are capable of better things doing what is expected of them but no more.'

Together they strenuously opposed state registration, which was sponsored by Mrs Bedford Fenwick who continued to advocate it week after week in the *British Journal of Nursing*, as the *Nursing Record* had now become. In this Miss Lückes and Knutsford had the backing of Miss Nightingale. According to Miss Lückes it would 'standardize mediocrity'. Miss Nightingale went further: it would 'degrade the high art of nursing to the status of a mere profession'. The matrons of many other hospitals also opposed it. Rivalry, they said, was best, and hospitals should compete in respect of the standards they could demand for their certificate. So, as a constructive alternative, Knutsford and Miss Lückes advocated an official nursing directory in which the qualifications of a woman as a nurse, and the hospital at which she had trained, would be stated.

The practical training of the probationers was delegated to the ward sisters, but matron arranged for certain others to help them with their studies during their off-duty period. The standard manual which they all read was, of course, her own. This, it will be remembered, had first been published as collected lectures. In 1889 she had rewritten it as a book, but it was something much more than a textbook, incorporating, as it did, all her high ideals of a nurse's attitude to her work and her patients. Nursing demanded a right sense of values as well as technical knowledge. That was Miss Lückes's thesis.

'There is a real danger at the present day that the fact that nursing is an art may be lost sight of, and that work which offers scope for the exercise of the best qualities of which human nature is capable may thus be degraded. Those who put their faith in examinations as a means of judging whether a woman possesses those qualities which alone can make her services acceptable in the sick room are no nearer solving the problem of getting the right type of woman. Technical knowledge is of secondary importance. It can never take the place of those characteristics which are essential to real nursing.'

14

Scientific Medicine

While Knutsford had been reconstructing the hospital and Miss Lückes revolutionizing the nursing, the modern medical college had been slowly taking shape.

This, in the first instance, seems to have been largely due to the vision of a surgeon, H. P. Dean, elected to the medical staff of the hospital in 1892; 'a tall, fine, upstanding man, with a large moustache of which he took great care', as Hugh Lett, a student then, describes him. 'He was a brilliant and progressive surgeon', continues Lett (later on the staff himself). 'He was also a pioneer in spinal anaesthesia, and I have vivid recollections of his classes in operative surgery. In his private practice his Spencer Wells forceps were gold-plated. In those very early days of motor cars he had two, and always took both when going to an operation. He drove one and, in case it broke down, his chauffeur followed behind in the other.'

Dean possessed other qualities besides those that had made him an outstanding surgeon. 'A man with the ability of a statesman,' wrote Arthur Keith, 'he resolved to reorganize the teaching in the School.' Hitherto all the best posts in the college had been held by physicians and surgeons to the hospital. Treves taught anatomy; Mansell Moullin, a physician, physiology; and Percy Kidd and Frederick Eve pathology. Dean now saw that anatomy was developing as a science on its own, and that modern physiology was essential to medical practice, while our knowledge of pathology was widening so fast that physicians and surgeons could no longer possibly keep pace with it. The vested interest of the staff of the hospital in these subjects must be broken, Dean saw, and the teaching of them handed over to specialists. How was this to be done?

His opportunity came when Mansell Moullin retired. Dean now succeeded in persuading the college board to appoint Leonard Hill, who had worked with Schafer in Edinburgh, to the lectureship in physiology. Then the demonstratorship in anatomy fell vacant and Dean saw that it was advertised in the public press. Arthur Keith decided to apply. 'I soon learnt that the man to help me was Dean, but rivalry had sprung up between him and Treves, and I was warned that, if I was backed by Dean, I would be opposed by Treves.' And it worked out just like that. Dean was encouraging. 'I was deeply impressed by his manifest ability.' Treves was curt. The proper person to teach anatomy, he said, was the surgeon. Then, when Keith had lost all hope, he got a note from James Galloway, a friend of Treves and a graduate of Keith's own university of Aberdeen. Galloway had been getting at Treves and now wrote to suggest that Keith should call on him a second time. Again Treves was curt but this time agreed to support him. So Keith got the job, and his foothold in the medical college.

He found it a strange place after Scotland. There the medical schools had started first and the hospitals been built up on them. In London it had been the other way round. With the exception of University College and King's – both nineteenth-century foundations – the hospitals had been founded first and their medical schools developed later. In consequence, as Keith found, there was a profound difference in hospital–medical school relationship south of the border. 'The high luminaries at "the London",' he wrote, 'were not the leaders of the Medical School [as they had been in Scotland] but the physicians and surgeons on the staff of the Hospital.' Nor was he happy in London at first. He was a comparative anatomist, both by training and inclination, and, handicapped by his Scottish accent and a natural lack of fluency, found teaching topographical anatomy to medical students difficult. When, however, Openshaw, the orthopaedic surgeon who had succeeded Treves as lecturer in anatomy, resigned, Keith was appointed in his place.

Pathology, literally the science of disease, had long been held synonymous with morbid anatomy. But people do not die of what can be seen in their bodies after they are dead, and other facets of pathology were now developing, notably bacteriology. Something had to be done now about the teaching of that. William Bullock, another Scot and an outspoken and stimulating person, and a great raconteur, was now appointed to teach it in the college, and soon attained notoriety – although it seems rather off his subject – by working out the inheritance of haemophilia in the royal family.

The college now paraded three remarkable personalities: Leonard Hill, Arthur Keith, and William Bullock. 'Many an interesting discussion did we have over lunch in the College dining-room,' writes Arthur Keith, 'especially when Head and Bullock came together' – for the former had joined the staff of 'the London' from University College, and was now maintaining the tradition for neurology at 'the London' started by Hughlings Jackson. He was much loved and respected by his patients, but his real interests were scientific. By studying the distribution of the rash in herpes zoster (shingles) and following cases of it to the post-mortem room, he succeeded in mapping out the surface of the body into skin areas according to the particular spinal root by which the sensory fibres from them enter the spinal cord. He got a surgeon to divide a sensory nerve in his own arm and, in conjunction with Rivers of St John's College, Cambridge, studied the return of sensation as the nerve regenerated. Among his other contributions to neurology was a series of papers on the sensory pathways in the brain and spinal cord, based on a follow-up to the post-mortem room.

Another frequent participant in these arguments was Harold Barnard, a nephew of Michael Faraday. He worked with Hill and together they invented, independently of and almost simultaneously with Riva-Rocci in Italy, the method which is used by every doctor today to measure his patient's blood pressure. This was a notable achievement in itself. They also used it on patients, and in fact introduced the measurement of blood pressure into medical practice. Barnard was only a registrar then. Later he became a distinguished member of the surgical staff.

The mechanism of the heartbeat at this date was attracting much attention. For the auricular–venticular bundle, strands of primitive tissue which conduct the stimulus to contract from the auricles to the ventricles, had been discovered. But where did this stimulus originate? All over the auricles simultaneously was one possibility; at one particular point in them, another. That was the problem that began to fascinate Arthur Keith and, in order to find out, he started to cut sections – for microscopic examination – of innumerable hearts, both animal and human. In every one of them he discovered, at the point known to comparative anatomists as the sino-auricular node, a remnant of primitive tissue. This seemed common to all animals, and Keith guessed that it must be the place where the stimulus to the heart beat originates. Five years later this guess was confirmed as fact, by means of the electrocardiograph.

One evening Keith happened to read a paper on irregularity of the heart, written by a certain James Mackenzie who was in general practice in Lancashire, and Keith wrote to him, explaining the reason for his interest in it. Mackenzie replied by return. He had the hearts, he said, of a number of his former patients who had died with – Mackenzie was careful not to say 'of' – some kind of cardiac irregularity. Would Keith see whether he could find any anatomical reason for it?

These hearts arrived in the medical college in the December of 1907, divided into two lots. The first contained those of patients who had exhibited occasional irregularity; the second were those of patients whose hearts had always been irregular, and in whom Mackenzie had inferred auricular paralysis on account of the invariable absence of any evidence of auricular activity in these patients during life, as judged from tracings taken from the great veins in their necks. In the first group Keith found nothing abnormal, confirming Mackenzie's view – contrary to that held by almost the entire medical profession at that date – that irregularity of this kind was of no particular significance. In the second,

Keith noticed that the auricles, which Mackenzie had imagined paralysed, were hypertrophied, i.e. unduly muscular, which was a complete contradiction in terms of biological law. How could paralysed muscle possibly become hypertrophied? There was only one way out of this dilemma. Their fibres must all be contracting, but contracting independently of each other with the result that there was no effective auricular beat. So, auricular fibrillation replaced the diagnosis of auricular paralysis. This concept was confirmed, like that of the origin of the heartbeat, by the electrocardiograph a few years later.

Mackenzie was now at the height of his reputation and, having migrated from Burnley to London, began to spend two afternoons a week working with Keith on the morbid anatomy of the diseased heart. Shortly after this, through Keith's influence, he was appointed lecturer in cardiology in the college. Then Knutsford, his eyes ever open to anything that would redound to the credit of 'the London', invited him to join the staff. A ward was allocated to his patients and a cardiac department started with Mackenzie at its head.

Morbid anatomy, particularly as studied under the microscope, was becoming increasingly important in many fields of medical research. So, in 1907, the pathology institute was enlarged and modernized, and handed over from the medical staff to Dr Salaman as full-time director, but the physicians and surgeons would still often come down to carry out post-mortem examinations themselves. This had long been their wont: again and again the post-mortem would confirm, elaborate or disprove a diagnosis made during life. Permission for as many post-mortems as possible was therefore always sought as the correlation of the findings in the body after death with the symptoms and signs exhibited by the patient during life was, and remains, an important facet in the art of diagnosis. Morbid anatomy, is in fact, basic to medical education, so the physicians and surgeons taught in the post-mortem room themselves.

Three years later Salaman retired and Hubert Turnbull, a student of 'the London' who had studied morbid anatomy in Germany, was appointed director in his place. He found himself

HUBERT MAITLAND TURNBULL, F.R.S.

RUSSELL HOWARD ON A TEACHING ROUND

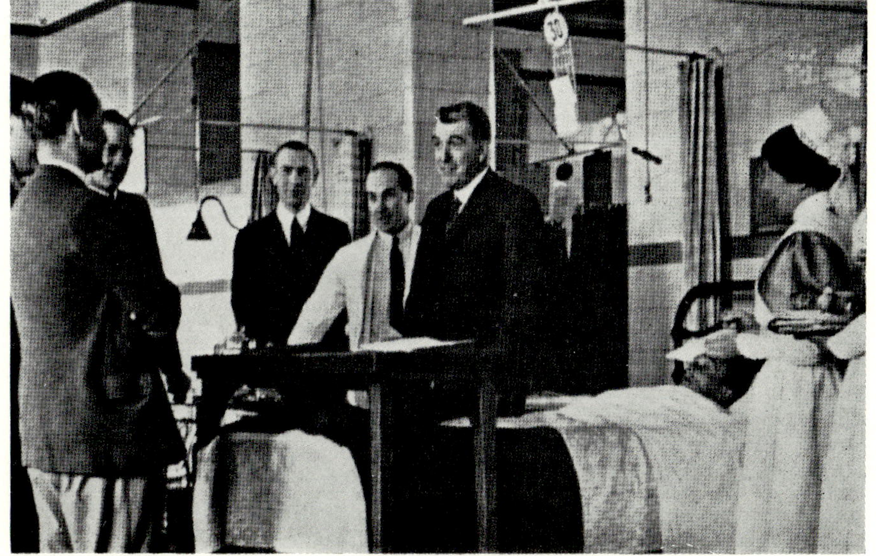

From left to right: Henry Thompson, J. W. Hannay, Russell Howard

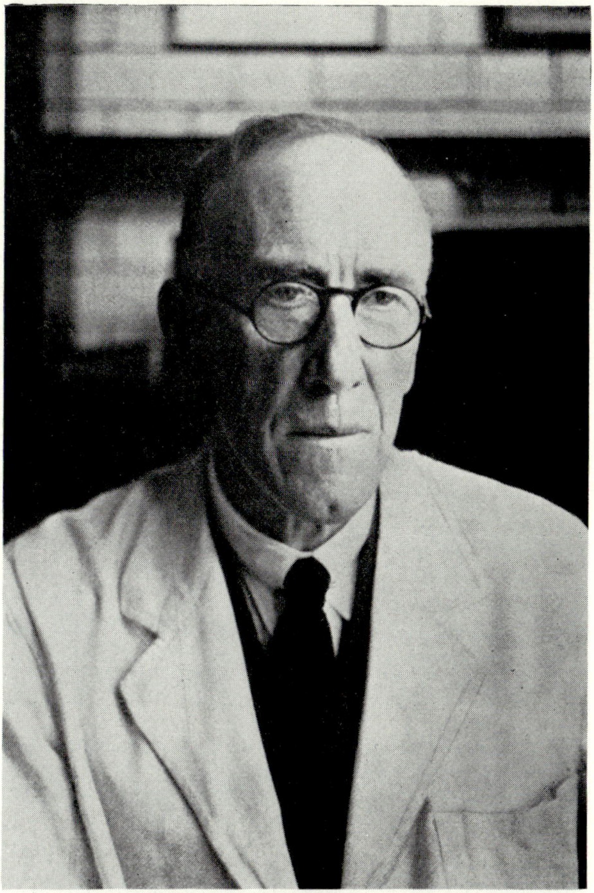

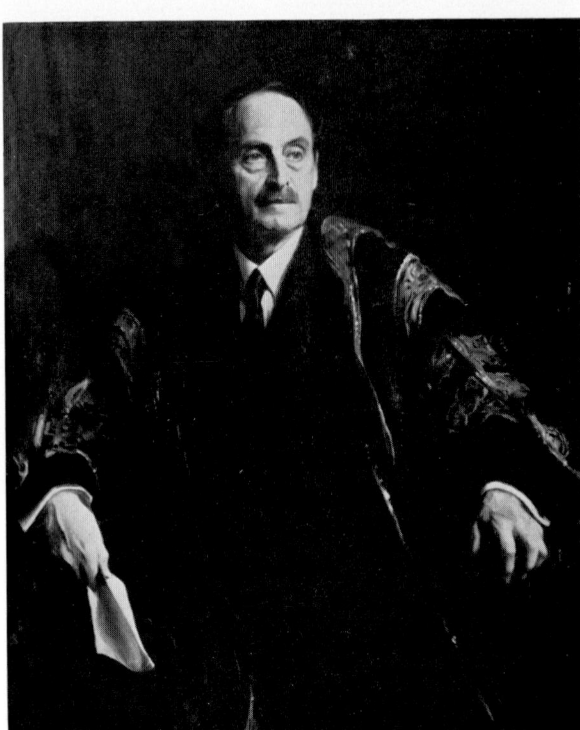

LORD DAWSON
The portrait by de Laszlo
(*Reproduced by permission
of the Royal College of
Physicians*)

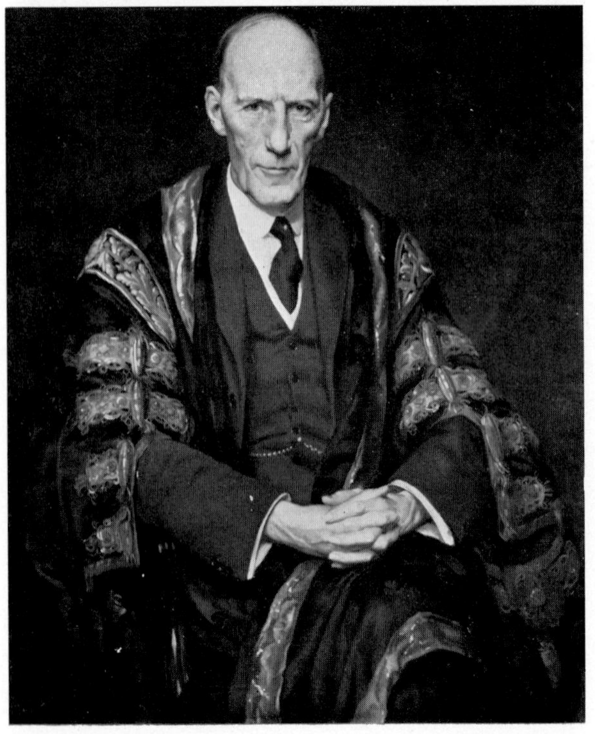

SIR ROBERT
HUTCHISON
The portrait by James
Gunn
(*Reproduced by permission
of the Royal College of
Physicians*)

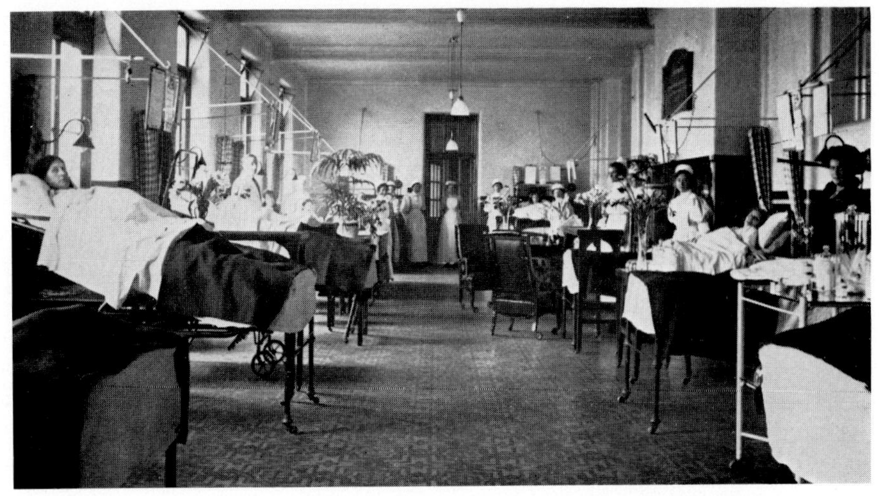

VICTORIA WARD

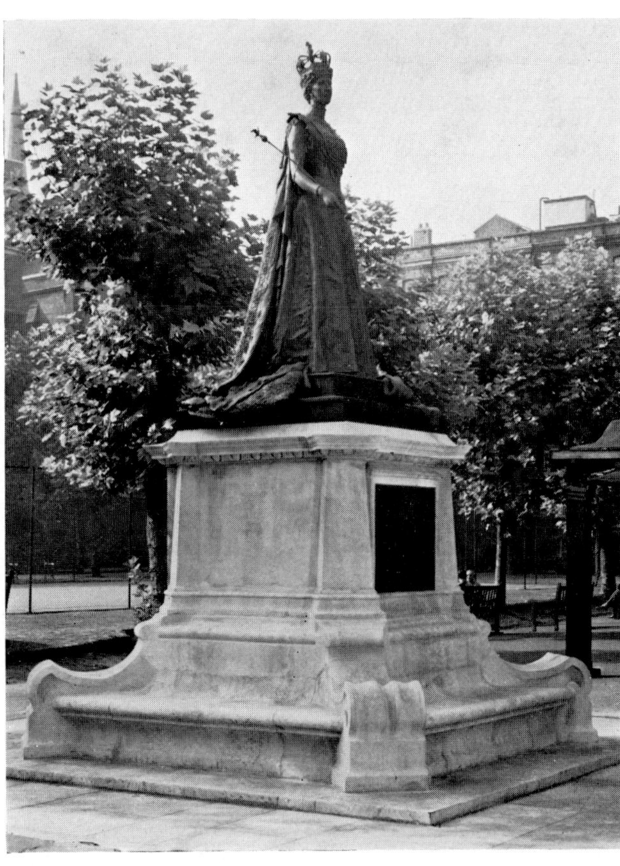

QUEEN ALEXANDRA
The statue by James
Wade erected in 1908

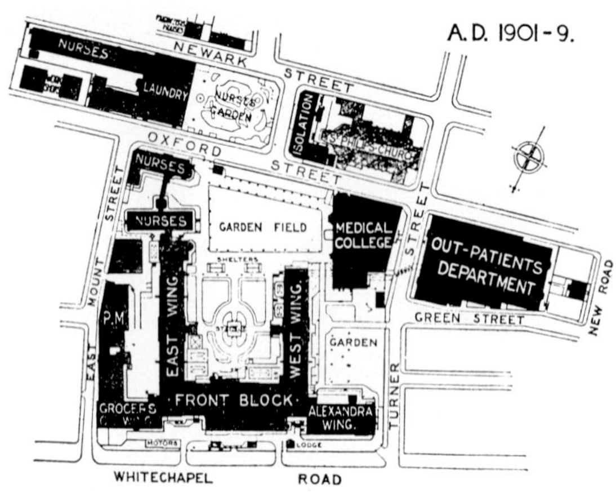

CHRISTMAS 1914

IN THE NEW OUT-
PATIENT DEPARTMENT
From left to right:
Sir Stephen MacKenzie,
Sir Frederick Treves,
Mr Sydney Holland,
Princess Victoria,
the King, the Queen,
the Duke of Cambridge,
the Bishop of Stepney,
the Bishop of London
(*From the Daily Graphic*)

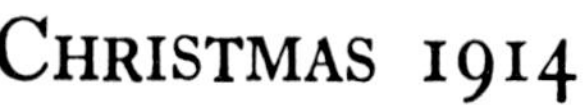

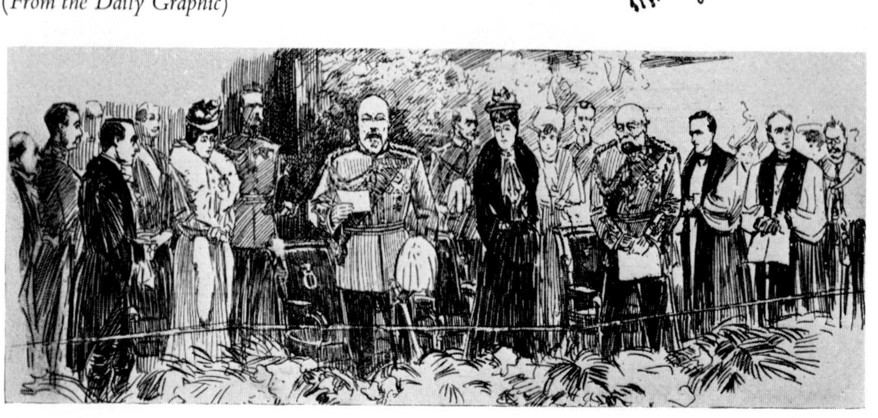

in a difficult position. The medical staff would arrive late. Their technique was haphazard. Again and again they 'spoilt the P.M.' Their observations were hurried and frequently inaccurate. This way of doing things, Turnbull saw, could be no serious basis for research. So, backed by Knutsford, who, although primarily interested in the immediate welfare of patients, had the vision to see the long-term importance of research, he secured agreement for all post-mortems to be performed in future by the director or one of his assistants. The whole body was now dissected in every case, routine observations faithfully recorded, and a collection of specimens, invaluable in almost every field of medicine, was rapidly built up. Further, Turnbull, with his infinite capacity for hard work, his flair for meticulous observation and his hatred of theory and speculation of any kind, had soon created a spirit of progress in his institute which came to dominate almost every other department of the hospital.

In 1900 the London Hospital Medical College had been incorporated as a school of the University of London (founded as an examing body in 1836) along with the other medical schools and University and King's Colleges. Not that this had made any immediate difference to it; the academic spirit had begun to invade the practical hospital-based medical school long before the turn of the century, and the college remained financially self-supporting in the sense that it paid the teachers' salaries and the rent of its premises, and bought materials and equipment, entirely out of its own income, derived in part out of a grant from the hospital in return for services rendered in kind, and in part out of students' fees. This change in fact was really, at that time, one of status only.

In the meantime Munro Scott, the ex-naval paymaster and warden of the college, had retired, in 1910, and been replaced by a dean responsible for the selection of students and the organization of medical education, and a secretary, responsible to the college board for finance and all domestic matters. Many still remember William Wright, the first dean in the modern era. He had been appointed lecturer in anatomy, in succession to Arthur Keith, and had gained notoriety by identifying bones dug up in the Tower as those of the little princes murdered by Richard III. Hill, Bullock and Wright were now declared professors, although their salaries were still paid in full by the self-supporting college.

Life in the hospital and college was now enlivened by a battle. A raid on a shop in Houndsditch by three men and a woman (who had come to live near it) was believed to be imminent and, when the police went to arrest them, Sergeant Bentley was shot dead and five other officers seriously wounded, three of them mortally. Two of the men and the woman got away. The third was wounded in the mêlée and died in a house in the Commercial Road. His body and that of the dead policeman, and that of one of the other policemen who died almost at once, were taken to the hospital where they lay side by side in the mortuary chapel. The wounded policemen were admitted to the wards. Then, a few days later, firing was heard in Sidney Street just east of the hospital. The police had tracked the gang to Martin's Mansions and, when they demanded admission, had been met by a volley. Sergeant Leeson, seriously wounded in the chest, was carried into the hospital.

Knutsford hurried out to the scene of action. 'Being the only person in a top hat I was taken for someone in authority, and had assumed this role, when whizz came a bullet which made me take cover.' The two men were shooting at everyone who came in sight. This went on for some time. Then Winston Churchill, Home Secretary, arrived, 'as a person of his temperament was bound to do'. Guardsmen were sent for from the Tower, and before long a battery of field artillery arrived, took up positions, and established an observation post on the hospital roof. For some hours shooting continued with little effect. 'There were a few flesh wounds among the attacking party', continues Knutsford, 'and a number of minor casualties among over-curious civilians. All were treated at "the London", but some only after a long wait For many of the residents, who had gone out to see the fun, got "interned" on the roof of the "Rising Sun" when the police pushed their cordon back to keep civilians out of danger.' Eventually the house caught fire and two shots were heard inside. The men had taken their own lives and, as soon as it was possible,

Knutsford went in with the firemen and police. They found two bodies charred out of recognition, the last of the casualties it would have been thought. Not so: one of the firemen was kneeling down close to Knutsford examining them, when a hearthstone from the room above fell on him through a hole in the floor, breaking his back.

Under the inspired leadership of Lord Knutsford – he had now succeeded to his father's title – 'the London', reconstructed, indeed, almost rebuilt, now stood at the zenith of its reputation and as financially solvent as an institution based on the voluntary contributions of the charitable could possibly expect. (There was no cause for any loss of faith as yet in the future of the voluntary system.) The staff of the hospital was distinguished with James Mackenzie and Henry Head at the top; that of the medical college was distinguished, too: Keith, Bullock, Turnbull, Hill. Nursing at 'the London' was now regarded as first class. Confidence and satisfaction reigned in so far as people shut their eyes to the clouds which kept blowing up on the international horizon: the Balkan war, the growing might of Germany, the naval race, Agadir, and now the murder of the Archduke, that hot July of 1914, in the Serbian town of Sarajevo.

A month later, at midnight on 4 August 1914, Britain was at war with Germany. In the words of Sir Edward Grey, Foreign Secretary, 'the lights had gone out all over Europe'. The nineteenth century, which had projected its ethos well into the twentieth, had come to an end overnight. Nothing was ever to be quite the same again.

15

First World War

In the turmoil that now ensued the hospital was faced with many difficulties. The number of nurses it could supply to the armed forces had been agreed, but no plans made for the provision of doctors, and the services were now appealing for medical personnel. All unessential work was suspended, and as many doctors as possible liberated at once. Forty-five members of the lay staff were also allowed to enlist. In the college, students near qualification carried on; the rest faded rapidly away. (There were no reserved occupations as in the Second World War.) 'Let's get out and have a crack at them before it's all over'; that was the spirit of the hour. Modern war could not, it was believed, possibly last long. Kitchener alone thought otherwise.

On the other side of the Channel events moved with startling rapidity and two days after Le Cateau – the blind collision – Knutsford, who had promised five hundred beds and been assured of ample notice being given before they were required, got a sudden message from the War Office. A hundred wounded were on their way to London. Could the hospital take them and also arrange their transport from Waterloo, as the Army Medical Department had no ambulances available? So he phoned the chairman of Lyons, a member of the house committee, and within an hour a fleet of fourteen of the firm's vans were ready.

While this operation was in progress another urgent message came from the War Office. Could the hospital take in a hundred and fifty more? The nursing staff worked all night putting up

extra beds in other wards to clear two more for soldiers. Then
not 150, for which the hospital had prepared, but 200 arrived, and
yet more beds had to be put up to cope with ordinary civilian
needs. A few weeks later Antwerp fell and the hospital took in
200 wounded Belgians, contrasting sadly with the cheerful
casualties from Mons. 'Dazed broken men,' wrote Knutsford,
'whose land had been destroyed, whose homes had been scattered,
few had more than the clothes they were wearing. One had the
latch keys of his business near Brussels. Another hugged a bayonet
which he had taken from a German soldier.'

Many of the senior staff left to serve full-time in the Army or
Navy: Bertrand Dawson to become consulting physician to the
Army; Leonard Hill to undertake research for the Royal Flying
Corps; Henry Souttar to command a field ambulance; Charles
Lindsay and George Neligan to serve in casualty clearing stations.
More junior doctors were soon given commissions as ships'
doctors or regimental medical officers. On one occasion the entire
medical staff threatened to join up, and Knutsford was forced to
intervene. Chaos reigned, many confused as to where their duty
lay. Then, as the concept of a short war quickly over petered
out, and the struggle settled down to entrenched attrition on the
Western Front, the need for some thought-out system of stag-
gering the recruitment of medical personnel became more and
more apparent.

Commissions in the RAMC and Naval Medical Service were
now given to many applicants at once, but instead of being called
up immediately, they were seconded for civilian work until their
service in one of the armed forces was actually needed. The
government also undertook to take not more than five doctors at
a time from 'the London', and promised to do their best to
replace them by older men, or men unfit for service, if they could.
These arrangements were on a voluntary basis; there was no
compulsory service of any kind for anybody as yet. The government also undertook to refuse commissions to all newly
qualified men until they had completed at least three months on
the house.

As the number of students in the college dwindled, the supply of newly qualified men available to hold appointments on the house began to dry up; so much so that before long the hospital was forced to seek recruits from elsewhere. The work of the hospital had become even greater than before. 'Old Londoners' returned; even former members of the staff came back. Young doctors, too, came over from the States, as the United States was not yet at war, and offered their help. Before long, too, the college board took the then revolutionary step of taking women as students and these, on qualification, were to be given appointments on the house just like the men.*

Prices soon started to rise as in the Napoleonic Wars. It now cost much more to feed both the patients and the staff. Wages also rose all round. Salaries had now to be paid to junior staff who, before the war, had been satisfied to serve the hospital solely in return for the opportunity to gain clinical experience; bonuses, too, had to be paid to lay workers in the lower income groups to match the rising cost of living. Then there were those on half pay serving with the forces, while full salaries had to be paid to those who had temporarily stepped in and were now doing their work. The cost of dressings and drugs had increased. Cod-liver oil, extensively used in the treatment of tuberculosis, now cost five times as much as it had done before; atropine fourteen times, and aspirin five times, as much. Subscriptions and donations started falling off in favour of charities directly connected with the war. At the end of the first full year, in spite of payment by the government for services rendered, the hospital stood over £14000 in debt.

---

* In 1888, Mrs Elizabeth Garrett Anderson (who before her marriage had been granted special permission to gain some experience of nursing at the hospital) had requested that women who wanted to become doctors should be able to train at 'the London'. The house committee had been 'prepared to view the proposal with favour, if it could be carried out without injury to the Hospital', but the medical staff came down heavily against it. 'We, the undersigned,' they wrote in a letter to the committee, 'are strongly of opinion that this measure would prove highly injurious to the interests of the Hospital and would probably lead to the break-up of the Medical School.' Then followed all their signatures with two exceptions, and they, as their active dissent is not recorded, were probably away at the time. The matter never seems to have been raised again. The view held at all the teaching hospitals was that a woman's proper vocation was nursing.

Many firms had difficulty in fulfilling their contracts, partly due to general shortage of labour, partly due to lack of raw materials due to government requisitioning, but the addition of two floors to Mr Fielden's isolation block, another gift from the Grocers' Company, was completed before the year was out; the nurses' home being built in East Mount Street was largely financed out of a fund raised by the *Daily Mirror*, and was completed in the following years. The latter, by request of Queen Alexandra, was now named the Cavell Home in memory of a London Hospital nurse who, on 12 October 1915, had been executed by a firing squad for helping British fugitives from Mons to escape from German-occupied Belgium.

Edith Cavell had joined the hospital as a pro in 1895 and, soon after gaining her London certificate, had gone out to Brussels to start a training school on British lines under Dr Depage. He was dissatisfied with Belgian nursing still in the hands of the Church. True to her training under Miss Lückes, with whom she continued to correspond, she had dedicated her life to raising the standard of nursing throughout the country. Now that Belgium had been overrun by the Germans an underground movement to help fugitive soldiers to escape, led by the Prince and Princess de Cröy, sought her help. Would she hide some British in her hospital until they could be got across the frontier into neutral Holland? They would be shot if she did not, she was told. Like a heroine in Greek tragedy she had, in fact, suddenly been caught up by events far outside her own control and forced into an impossible position, forced by her own conscience into a course of action which would risk the school under her charge, and wreck her ideals of better nursing in Belgium. She agreed – how could she have done otherwise? – and was gradually drawn deeper and deeper into this escape organization until she became an organizer herself. Soon it was discovered, many arrests were made, and the conspirators tried by a military court. Edith Cavell and Philippe Baucq, a Belgian architect, were condemned to death and others, including the Princess – the Prince escaped in time – sentenced to hard labour. Her execution proved a political blunder of the highest order although on legal grounds the Germans were fully justified in what they did. Under the guise of nursing she had given assistance to their enemies.

The first of Count Zeppelin's dirigible airships crossed the North Sea in January 1915, and in the late summer 'Zep' raids on outer London on moonlight nights became fairly frequent:

> Hail to thee, high flier,
> Who with generous heart
> Pourest out thy fire
> Over earth's dim chart
> In sundry spasms of well-premeditated art!
>
> O'er thy bloated carcass
> Plays the silver beam,
> Where, in azure darkness, as
> In a nightmare's dream,
> Thy crew are swung, and wish themselves elsewhere, I deem.
>
> Forth from many a tile (hark!)
> Boom the happy guns,
> Having quite a sky-lark
> Blazing at the Huns,
> With now a decent shot, and now some rotten ones.
>
> Didst thou look for panic,
> Counting on a scare
> Caused by that Titanic
> Sausage up in air?
> Then let me tell thee, London hasn't turned a hair.
>
> With the morrow's dawning,
> Rose, and all serene,
> Turned – a little yawning –
> To the day's routine,
> And went about her work as if thou hadst not been.*

No bombs ever fell near the hospital but on two occasions watchers from the windows saw a Zeppelin caught in the intersecting beams of searchlights and come down in flames.

When I got back to England in the autumn of 1916 the shadow

* Owen Seamen, *To a Zeppelin*, reprinted by permission of *Punch*.

of the Somme and the mounting German U-boat campaign had fallen over England's green and pleasant land. The cry of 'business as usual', with the regular army doing the fighting, a catch phrase at the beginning, had long ceased to be heard. The concept of a war quickly over had faded out of mind. No end to it now seemed in sight. Casualties had rendered the manpower problem desperate. Kitchener's volunteers and Lord Derby's scheme had failed to close the ranks; conscription had been introduced.

The medical college was a shadow of its former self. There cannot have been eighty students in it altogether, and many, like myself, were ex-combatants released, now that conscription was in force, to make good, in due course, the increasing deficiency of doctors in the services. William Wright was still dean, but we clinical students saw little of him. Our lives were guided by the secretary, E. J. Burdon, a frail, hard-working, helpful little man (who always wore a high, stiff, white collar and had a nervous habit of gulping in his throat), assisted by Osman, the registration clerk, a little dark square man of Turkish extraction and a friend at court to countless generations of 'old Londoners'.

Theodore Thompson, a man of outstanding intellectual ability, taught us medicine. He had already worked with Head on the classification of sensory impulses in the spinal cord, and his clinical interests were in a wide field. He had a large private practice, so large that his classes were often lamentably curtailed by his late arrival. 'He was known as the Turtle,' wrote Lord Brain, 'on account of his rotund build and somewhat rolling gait, and this appearance was accentuated by the fact that he usually wore a tail coat.' My surgical firm was Hutchinson (the son of his great father) and Warren. The former was learned, but clinically unimpressive. It was Richard Warren, who stood and walked like the boxer that he was, who went out of his way to teach us. He also came down every night, when the firm was on full duty, to do the emergency operations.

F. J. Smith, now a colonel in the R A M C, carried on his routine visits to 'the London' and always kept his military cap on when going round the wards. (I can see him now, with the cap on the back of his head, leaning over a patient, with his stethoscope in his ears.) Although the kindest of men he tended to be crude and his remarks, though often to the point, were sometimes an embarrassment to sister, who would turn her back and walk away. His medical knowledge was not profound. I never heard any original remarks fall from his lips, but he was a good hack teacher. So, too, was Russell Howard, that is, if you liked his style. He bullied us into knowledge, and some were frightened of being made to look fools. I soon discovered how important it was to stand up to him.

Most impressive were Robert Hutchison and Head. The former, the dry Scot, said little, but every word he did say was worth hearing, and many of his pronouncements became famous. 'Like a vegetarian, full of wind and self-righteousness', is typical of his caustic remarks. His medical 'litany' ought to be read still. One verse must suffice to indicate its style. 'From making the treatment worse than the disease, good Lord deliver us.' He was a brilliant diagnostician and continued to ignore X-rays. In the summer he lectured on therapeutics; not that there was much therapeutics in those days, but his lectures were worth listening to for the sheer elegance of his diction, which matched his own tall, erect figure in that long, grey frock coat. Henry Head, on the other hand was talkative and histrionic, his public demonstration the bright spot of the students' working week.

Miss Lückes was still matron, and continued to take a deep personal interest in all her nurses. I can see her now in her habitual black satin and little white lace cap, with rings on her fingers and jewellery on her dress. She was now crippled with rheumatism and an imposing cortège would often pass through a ward. The door would be flung open suddenly. All eyes would turn in that direction. (Some degree of acting is essential to command.) Then a pause before a uniformed porter appeared pulling, and behind him, in her wheelchair, the little old lady, looking like Queen Victoria, and behind her another porter pushing, and, bringing up the rear, her faithful maidservant, Hetty, bearing her habitual cushion and hot-water bottle. She would bow right and left as the procession moved down the ward until, half-way perhaps, it might halt and she would beckon some junior pro towards her.

'Tell me, nurse, about that patient – he looks very ill.' Then, satisfied on that point, the cortège would move on.

There were now two maternity charities. The white, run by the students, dating from 1863, and the green, run by the nurses, started by Miss Lückes in 1905. Four of us were detailed as 'midder boys' each month, and divided out time between the 'midder house' in Philpot Street, where we slept and fed, and the 'midder room' in the hospital, where a map of the district had been drawn on one of the walls by Henry Souttar. We went out to each case alone but, if we ran into difficulties, we could send a messenger up to the hospital with a 'flag' for the junior resident accoucheur, who would come and help. Many of my patients could only speak Yiddish, German written in Hebrew characters, and the district ranged from Bethnal Green and Shoreditch in the north to Ratcliffe Highway, Wapping and London Docks in the south. So I got some idea of the squalor under which the population of East London still lived. I delivered twenty-eight women in a month and, as we had to visit each mother three times after her baby was born, I was soon getting very little sleep. It also involved much travelling, which we did on bicycles.

In this gloomy year German aeroplanes first dropped bombs on London. On 13 June 1916 I was in the out-patient department at about 11 a.m. when an explosion shook the building, and I got outside just in time to see seven aeroplanes – they were not flying high – silhouetted against the clear blue morning sky. This bomb had fallen near by, and others were dropped in the vicinity of Aldgate. Before long casualties were streaming in. They came in ambulances, tradesmen's vans and hand-carts, or were carried on stretchers and shutters: 207 arrived in the space of less than an hour. A bus that had been hit drove straight to the hospital with its casualties on board. Serious cases were rushed up to the wards, and before long the receiving room was full and a line of stretchers blocked the main corridor, house surgeons and dressers going round giving morphine and anaesthetics to those in severe pain. Seventy-five casualties were taken in. Forty-four died. Thirty were brought in dead.

No other daylight raiders got very near the hospital and, as the

British anti-aircraft defences improved, daylight gave way to moonlight bombing. At the end of September a spell of brilliant weather combined with a full moon enabled the Germans to keep London under fire for several nights in succession and before long (unlike their reaction to the much more severe blitz of the last war), a section of the population of the East End was reduced to a state bordering on panic and the hospital was faced with a serious problem. On likely nights, or as soon as the maroons went off (there were no sirens in those days, and, aeroplanes flying slowly, the period of warning before the raid started was much longer), thousands of the inhabitants of Whitechapel would seek shelter in the basement. 'The jam in the passage on the first occasion was terrific,' writes Knutsford, 'but one late arrival contrived to bore his way through to the safest point. He was a little man, but he pushed before him an enormously stout lady and each time he piped out "maternity case" won another foot or two of ground.' The smell of unwashed humanity would permeate the whole building, and this overcrowding was potentially dangerous as, in the event of fire, it would have proved impossible to work the hydrants. So before long admission was limited to women and children and the gates were closed after 2000 had come in.

The work of the hospital continued. No wards were closed, and the theatres on the top floor remained in use even when a raid was in progress, for these night raids never assumed the serious proportions of those in the second war. Few raiding planes got through, and their bombs were of low explosive power, but on the night of 19 January 1917 London was shaken by a shattering explosion. Four tons of TNT had blown up at the munition works at Silvertown two miles east of the hospital, devastating a square mile of surrounding houses. A sinister yellow glow suffused the eastern horizon, so bright that it was possible to read a paper in the street. The house governor's staccato report gives a vivid impression of the hospital that night. '6.50 p.m. a terrific explosion, quite unlike anything we had had before and which made the whole building sway, followed immediately by people running and calling, the sound of falling glass and the smell of burning. (231 Hospital windows had been broken; the latter due to soot falling down the chimneys.) No reply from exchange! Rumours flying round! Stepney gas works, Limehouse powder works, Woolwich Arsenal? Then Poplar rang. They were dealing with a hundred casualties and would send the rest on to us. Arbour Square police station could give no information. Then Canning Town rang. Enormous explosion. Short of doctors. Could we send? Got five men and three women into a cab with dressings, chloroform and instruments. But driver "wasn't going to Canning Town for anybody." Took his number and got another. Gentleman in car 10 miles away drove straight to hospital and picked up dressings and dressers. Then Canning Town rang again. How many casualties could we take? Replied up to three hundred if necessary. So got 100 extra beds put up in an hour. Office sisters worked like niggers. Soon every ward full and spare beds down corridors. Injured now started coming up in motor lorries, carts and carried on shutters and doors. Took in 60 and housed many homeless. Four died during the night. One child of eight arrived with baby in her arms and leading another of four. Couldn't find her mother and had been picked up by lorry driver in devastated street. Bitterly cold admitting cases but hot coffee doled out in gallons to drivers, police, porters and others. Admitted one woman badly injured whose seven children had been killed. Little dog came up with a fearfully injured woman and wouldn't leave her. So we let it go into the ward with her. The taxi now returned. But they could do nothing. They had never seen such a sight. A square mile blazing. Heat fearful and there must be hundreds buried. No good waiting. All very much upset but had stopped to help at Poplar on the way back. No more cases admitted. This morning, Saturday, very sad work. Relatives searching for relatives. All buried I am afraid. One woman said she had seen forty loads of dead bodies taken off somewhere today.'

I qualified in January 1918 and was appointed house physician to two men of very different type, although each one, in his own way, typified so many who have served 'the London'. Wilfred Hadley was an aloof and frightening personality who used to shout at me and my inexperience down the telephone, almost inaudible on account of the cigar between his teeth. Lewis Smith was genial, kindly, helpful, and full of good advice. 'You will make lots of mistakes,' he said to his new housemen, 'but don't take acute osteomyelitis into one of my beds and call it acute rheumatism.' Hadley, after he had been round, had the diagnosis of every patient taped. Few felt much better. He had said and done too little. True, there were no medical therapeutics then that really accomplished much but, after Lewis Smith's rounds, people invariably felt better. He always had a word to say to everyone, and always made a show of doing something, ordering this here, altering that prescription there. On the other hand, again and again he had not got a clue as to the diagnosis of a case. Nevertheless, or rather, perhaps it is easily understandable that he was in high demand in the East End as a consultant in those days. It was invaluable experience, but on 21 March Ludendorff launched his final attack against the British. I had still another month on the house but, with all my contemporaries, I was called up for service in the RAMC immediately.

Germany had shot her bolt. Her onslaught was held, and by November it was clear that the war would soon be over. Then, at this juncture, as if Europe had not endured enough already, the first great wave of influenza started sweeping across it from the East. There had been an epidemic of a mild kind during the summer; this second edition of it was a very different thing. A high proportion of cases developed broncho-pneumonia within a few days, or even a day, of the first onset of symptoms. During the week ending 21 October, of fifty-five cases admitted, over 50 per cent died, and a week later an emergency meeting reviewed the very serious position with which the hospital was faced. There had been nothing like it since the cholera! Again the hospital was being asked to admit many more cases than it could take with the number of beds and reduced nursing staff (the latter a consequence of the epidemic itself) at its disposal. Further, the disease was highly contagious and, although now universal, some attempt at segregation was clearly necessary. Wards were set aside for 'flu cases, and by the end of December 1918, 140 cases had been admitted, of whom 96 died, although the hospital did not lose a single nurse. Then the disease waned but burst out again with renewed violence in February of the new year when three nurses and eighty more patients died in the hospital. The epidemic had been much worse than that of 1889–90. In the United Kingdom alone it led to the deaths of 200000 people. In the world at large it is said to have killed millions.

Meanwhile, the long weary war had been drawing to an end at last, and at the eleventh hour of the eleventh day of the eleventh month in its fifth year, bugles sounded the cease-fire over the whole Western Front. In London the maroons went off and the pent-up emotion of four years of war, and of those daily casualty lists (the horror of which those who have only known the Second World War can but dimly appreciate), was let loose. In Whitehall and the West End every one rushed out into the street. In the hospital the menace of influenza was forgotten. Patients jumped out of bed and crowded the balconies. Classes and lectures broke up in confusion. Nurses off duty rushed into the garden. All wanted to share the relief of it with others, and with as many as they could.

16

Financial Struggle

The war had left all the hospitals heavily in debt. Prices and wages had risen; the cost of treating patients increased. At 'the London' the deficit on the last year of it alone amounted to over £65000 and, even if legacies now continued to fall in at average level, subscriptions, it was clear, would need to rise by at least a hundred per cent if it was to remain solvent.

Something had to be done about it, and the house committee decided to recommend a step which had long been in their minds. Patients who could afford it should, they thought, now be asked to make some contribution towards their keep. This would be no infringement, as they saw it, of the voluntary system. The spirit of that would still be maintained. Social conditions had changed. The East End was no longer quite the same place of squalor and destitution. The working classes were now better off and under the Insurance Act of 1912 the working man's income no longer wilted right away as soon as he came into hospital.

Many people were, however, wondering whether the voluntary system was not really doomed. Others, even then, would have welcomed government assistance with corresponding government control. So a committee was set up by the Ministry of Health (which had now replaced the Local Government Board) under the chairmanship of Lord Cave. Is the voluntary system worth saving? they were asked. Their reply was categorical. 'We are convinced that it is. If it fails, then the hospitals must be provided by the public, and the expense will be enormous. But the monetary loss to the state would be small compared to the injury done to the sick, the training of doctors, and the progress of research. That personal relationship between patient, doctor and nurse, often making the time spent in a hospital ward the happiest period of a patient's life, would be difficult to maintain under an official régime. Nor is the educational site of the present system less important. Medical education in this country is still to a large extent a private enterprise. The voluntary hospital system, which is peculiar to the English-speaking people, is part of the heritage of our generation and it would be lamentable if, by our apathy or folly, it were suffered to fall into ruin.'

The hospitals of this country, the Cave Committee said – they seem to have largely ignored the workhouse infirmaries – should continue to rely on charity. Subscriptions, legacies and bequests, they believed, supplemented by payments by patients who could afford to contribute towards their keep, as had now been started at 'the London', and insurance schemes against hospital charges, as were already under consideration elsewhere, would be sufficient to maintain them. As, however, many of the hospitals required some immediate assistance in consequence of the war, they recommended a grant in aid of a million pounds and a commission to administer it.

Meanwhile another committee had been sitting. For Dawson, now senior physician to 'the London', had given his Cavendish lectures on *The National Welfare – the future of the Medical Profession*, as the result of which Dr Christopher Addison, the first Minister of Health, had set up a 'Consultative Committee on medical and allied services' under Dawson's chairmanship with Ernest Morris, the house governor of 'the London', as one of its members. Their terms of reference were to plan a medical service for the whole country. In May 1920 they had submitted an interim report. Primary health centres staffed by general practitioners, they recommended, should be set up throughout the country based on secondary centres in the larger towns staffed by specialists. The latter were to be affiliated to the teaching hospitals.

The short-lived post-war boom was over by this time however, retrenchment was in the air, and all plans involving expenditure

G

were now mercilessly axed. The grant to the voluntary hospitals, recommended by Lord Cave's committee, was halved. Nothing came of the recommendations of the Dawson report, but the committee over which he had presided, and which he had inspired, had been the first body of any kind to focus public attention on the need for an organized health service, and Lloyd George submitted his name for a peerage, the first in the profession since Lord Lister's. The Prime Minister wanted a real authority on health matters in the House of Lords. Dawson now became the recognized leader of the medical profession.

Meanwhile, in spite of the optimism of Lord Cave's committee, the governors of 'the London' had been forced into taking a step which had never been taken since the hard times of the Napoleonic wars. They felt compelled to close wards to the extent of a loss of over 200 beds, and this at a time when the list of semi-urgent cases waiting for admission stood at over a thousand! This was fully exploited by Knutsford in order to raise money for the hospital.

A considerable increase in subscriptions and two large donations followed. An American gave £5000 towards a new gynaecology theatre and promised another £5000 if £10000 more could be raised in other quarters. Here the Cave Commissioners stepped in, and the full benefit of Mr Bader's generosity was secured. The trustees of Sir William Dunn's estate also gave the hospital £5000 for the conversion of the clinical theatre above the front gate into new laboratories.

The Cave Committee had recommended a joint appeal to the public on behalf of all the voluntary hospitals. So, throughout 1922, Knutsford was forced to keep silent and this appeal lacked his personal touch. Certainly 'the London's' share of the money raised fell far short of what the hospital would have got if he had been allowed to appeal on behalf of his own hospital in his own inimitable style. The same year also proved an unfortunate one in respect of legacies and ended with a deficit of £18000. The financial outlook now looked a little more promising, however, and Knutsford, banking on this and 'the London's' own quinquennial appeal in the following year, persuaded the governors to reopen three of the closed wards, and to give up the X-ray department (above the front gate) and convert the basement of the Grocers' Wing (now Richmond ward but closed) for that purpose.

Knutsford's optimism proved justified. His quinquennial appeal next year exceeded all expectations. 'I have just had an outstanding offer made to me,' he wrote to the press when the appeal had already been running for nine months, 'such as I have never had before in my whole career.' He then went on to relate how an acquaintance (who had lived near the hospital for some years) had offered to double any gift to it before the end of the year, only limiting his liability in this respect to £80000! Thus began the great doubling appeal. Day by day the total grew, with a rush at the start, then slowly, then again more rapidly as closing time loomed near. As the final days ebbed out, excitement mounted. 'It was the sporting side of the appeal,' wrote Knutsford, 'the fight against probability and time – would the full £160000 be garnered in – and the stupendous generosity of the offer which caught the public fancy. On the last night before the last day only £3362 was needed to win and, when the next morning's post came in, I had never in my whole life seen such a sight! It was a beggar's dream! Over four thousand envelopes on the table (every one containing money) which, averaged at a reasonable figure, would cover the balance we needed twelve times over. When this sum had been reached, there were still two thousand envelopes unopened!' Then came a telegram from Sir Henry Mallaby-Deeley (of 30s. made-to-measure suit fame) offering to make good any deficit. Whereupon Knutsford wired back, would Sir Henry double the remaining unopened gifts instead? 'Up to a liability limited to £10000', came back the answer. This target was also reached. So the great doubling appeal brought £180000 into general funds. Knutsford had enjoyed every moment of it and, for the time being, the financial situation had been saved.

Meanwhile, there had been many changes on the staff, as I discovered when I got back to the hospital in the summer of 1920. Miss Lückes had died. Her successor, Miss Monk, had a reputation as a good business woman and was a sound administrator but lacked the personality of her predecessor. Nor did she understand the young. At a time when there was a growing shortage of nurses, largely due to the emancipation of women and to so many new ways of earning a living having become open to them, some relaxation of the Victorian attitude to the kind of life a nurse should lead was clearly demanded, but under her jurisdiction the idea of it as one of absolute dedication died hard. Nurses and sisters were still required to live in one of the three homes and, if one got engaged to a doctor, she was expected to leave the hospital at once. Excursions out with a student were still looked upon askance. Knutsford might well have been wiser to have brought back some successful 'London' and Lückes-trained matron from one of the provincial hospitals. There were now many of them. He was getting old, however, and may well have become fixed in his ideas.

Science was growing even faster into medical practice now. Medical and surgical 'units' with full-time staff, I found, had been started, as at some other teaching hospitals, along the lines recommended by the Haldane Commission on medical education. The idea of them hailed from Germany, where the university professor dominated medical practice in the hospital, and had been carried to the Johns Hopkins Hospital in Baltimore by the American bacteriologist Welch (he had spent the formative years of his life in Germany) and thence to England by Osler when appointed Professor of Medicine at Oxford. It was Osler who had urged on the Commission that a professor of medicine needed both a team of assistants and adequate laboratory facilities if he were to treat his patients properly, teach students as they should be taught, and advance medicine by research. So the Haldane Commission had persuaded the University Grants Committee (a department of the Privy Council) to put up the necessary money for teaching hospitals to try the 'unit' experiment if they wished.

Charles Miller, who had served as a consultant physician to the army during the war, had been persuaded to become first director of this new medical 'unit', and I was appointed his house physician. He was popular and, both in physical appearance and attitude to life, a typical John Bull. He was also a good clinician, but in no sense did he cut an academic figure. That deficiency in his make-up was made good by his two principal assistants; Arthur Ellis, a Canadian whose approach to clinical medicine had been from the laboratory, and George Riddoch, a brilliant Aberdonian, who had done important work on spinal injuries during the war. A disciple of Henry Head, he was now maintaining the tradition for neurology at 'the London' started by Hughlings Jackson in the nineteenth century.

My life on the 'unit' was strenuous. All three of my chiefs, unlike all other members of the staff who gave their professional services to the hospital for nothing, were full-time, salaried, and debarred from private practice. So they were always all in the house and, if I was not on some formal round, I always seemed to be with one of them examining and discussing a patient. Never, except at week-ends, did I seem to find time to examine and write up new cases until after nine at night! Nor can I remember taking a week-end off. Nor were house officers paid in those days: we were only too willing to do the work merely to gain experience. Many cases of post-vaccinial encephalitis (due to first vaccination at school age) were being admitted. Encephalitis lethargica was also common. This disease had spread across Europe from Austria during the last year of the war. I can see those cases of it now, lying in bed in semi-coma with drooping eyelids due to ocular paralysis. Soon after, it faded out as mysteriously as it had started.

As time went on and medicine progressed – insulin in the treatment of diabetes and liver extract in that of pernicious anaemia were discovered round about this time – more and more space per bed began to be required for X-rays, laboratories and secretaries. So the wards still closed were never reopened and, although the hospital still maintained over 800 beds, it never reverted to being as large in the strictly bed sense as it had been before the war. The perfection of the motor ambulance had, however, rendered country convalescent homes a practical proposition. This materially increased the rate of turnover of patients in the wards.

A new boilerhouse was built and oil fuel introduced. An out-patient VD department was started in collaboration with the LCC. Ultra-violet light treatment was provided for surgical tuberculosis. A massage department was opened by the Duke of Kent. But in the main Knutsford remained cautious about any major schemes demanding heavy capital outlay, for organized labour had become a political force and in November 1925 public opinion had swung sufficiently far to the left to put a Labour government, dependant on Liberal support, in office. At the next election an absolute Labour majority was possible. In that event increased taxation of the rich would follow, and this would affect subscriptions to all the voluntary hospitals adversely.

There had been minor strikes, but it was not until April 1926 that the great coal strike began. Then, on 3 May, when the miners had already been out some weeks, the TUC called a general strike in their support. Trains, trams and buses stopped running. New patients could not get to hospital to take up the beds; diabetics to get their essential insulin; non-resident staff to their work. Organized research was interrupted. I was working in the laboratory at the time, and when I turned on the electricity and nothing happened, I took myself off and functioned as lowest grade in a loco shed on the Midland Railway. (Had the strike lasted longer I might have been promoted to the footplate!) Students, too, faded away to help maintain essential services. That was the mood of the hour. Finsen light and X-ray treatment both had to be shut down, and after two days the out-patient department was closed. Knutsford, however, sought a personal interview with the Electrical Trade Union and they agreed to allow the labour necessary to restore electricity to the hospital.

The general strike, although it only lasted a week, had hit the hospital hard. The accounts for 1926 showed a deficit of nearly thirty thousand pounds in spite of the fact that by exercising extreme economy expenditure had been cut by several thousand. In the following year the situation was eased by legacies, and in 1928 Knutsford was able to launch his quinquennial appeal. 'I have been silent for five years,' he wrote to the press and repeated over the air in '*The London*' *calling*, the first broadcast of its kind (the BBC had just begun), 'and now once again I ask everyone to help the London Hospital. Somehow we simply must raise £250000. We have good cause enough. The largest hospital in England has been almost entirely rebuilt in the last thirty years at a cost of nearly one million pounds, and never in its 188 years of work for the poor has it been better able to fulfil its responsibilities. But here is the tragedy. Every year we have to face a large deficit. So far we have only succeeded in meeting these deficits by super efforts at our quinquennial appeals. I do not ask that the Hospital be made rich. I do ask that it should be made safe, if only as a tribute to the work it has done for the country.'

Over twenty thousand people responded to his words, written and across the air, which, as someone said, 'possessed a quality of faith which could hardly fail to touch the public's heart'. £26000 was brought up to the hospital that day, yet the total sum collected fell far below the target set. Money was too short; the future too uncertain; too many other charities were appealing to the public at the same time. Only £120000 resulted. Further, legacies were down that year, after the previous bumper one in that respect, while expenditure had risen by over £25000 due to repairs and renovations which had now become absolutely necessary as the result of the excessive economies of the past few difficult years. In 1929 things picked up a little. A credit balance of £20000, largely due to legacies, now enabled Knutsford to risk starting a radiotherapy department in the old boilerhouse and re-equiping the radiodiagnostic department. Then came the great depression of the thirties and, as luck would have it, a year lean in respect of legacies. Subscriptions fell off sharply. 'The full effect of the money stringency has yet to be faced,' wrote Knutsford in his report to the governors, 'and we must regard the future with considerable anxiety.'

He was not to be called upon to continue the unequal struggle much longer. On 5 July 1931 he was taken ill at his home and brought to the hospital. James Walton operated for acute intestinal obstruction, and he was soon well on his way to complete recovery, running the hospital from his bed, his mind full of plans as to how to use his illness, and rapid recovery, to the full as a way of raising yet more money for it. Then, just as all was set for him to go home, he had a sudden heart attack and died. The news spread rapidly. 'When the Hospital flag was hoisted at half mast,' writes his biographer, 'and silence fell on the great building, an incredible serenity seemed to permeate the wards and corridors and extend its influence right out into the busy street.'

'What would the London Hospital have been without Lord Knutsford?' wrote *The Times* next day. 'What, again, would the voluntary hospital system of this country be without the influence which from "the London", he exerted on it? Our hospitals have served the world for a model, and no man wrought with such selfless zeal or with such conspicuous success to make that model perfect as did the great Chairman of "the London".'

He had expressed the wish that no formal memorial should be raised in his memory, so a fund was started to be applied to the completion of the many additions and improvements to the hospital on which he had set his heart. In the end, however, the house committee decided that some memorial to so great a man must be erected somewhere. A tablet was designed by Lutyens and placed in the front hall above the main entrance so that the many who passed that way might read it:

> *A friend of all manner of men he will be remembered for his compassion for the sick and distressed. To them he gave the best of his powers. Rich beyond most men in the gifts of energy, courage and humour, he drew others to give with a sympathy and generosity akin to his own. Through him the Hospital was largely rebuilt and equipped to serve generations to come. Above all he inspired it in every part with his own spirit and love of service.**

'We have to remember how swiftly life changes,' said Sir William Goschen, his successor, at the unveiling ceremony, 'and the time will come when those who worked here with him will pass on and the traditions of the place will rest in other hands. It

---

* When the front hall was reconstructed this tablet was removed to an inferior position on the west wall of the entrance from the garden.

is for future generations that we have thought fit to have this memorial erected. We want all who follow to derive the same inspiration from his memory as we who worked with him derived from his arresting personality.'

17

Shadow of Another War

Knutsford's death coincided with a turning-point in the history of the voluntary hospitals. In spite of the findings of the Cave Committee it had become clear that they were unable to provide for all the acute sick. So Neville Chamberlain, Minister of Health in Stanley Baldwin's government, had introduced his Local Government Bill. The Boards of Guardians were abolished and the poor-law infirmaries handed over to the county councils to be converted into hospitals, although they remained under statutory obligation to provide for the destitute. The voluntary hospitals continued to take in most of the acute sick, but a higher and higher proportion of non-urgent cases, particularly those who could not afford to contribute towards their keep, started to gravitate towards these new county council hospitals. When Knutsford died, only about thirty per cent of the patients in 'the London' were being cared for entirely free. The rest contributed towards their keep according to their means.

Knutsford's death also coincided with a turning point in the history of the West. The hopes of a new era of peace and prosperity had been dashed. The drift towards another war had begun. His death, too, had also coincided with the financial crisis of the thirties. There had been heavy selling on the American stock market in 1929. This had affected trade the world over; in 1930 British exports had dropped by fifty per cent and unemployment risen to $2\frac{1}{2}$ million. Three days, in fact, after Knutsford's death the May Report anticipated a deficit of 132 million pounds at the end of the financial year, and taxation was raised, and salaries and pay cut, to meet the enormous cost of unemployment benefit. In spite of this the value of the pound slumped and Britain was forced off the gold standard.

Goschen had taken over at a difficult moment. At the end of his first full year as chairman, and in spite of a reduction of £12000 in running costs brought about by an economy drive in every department of the hospital, he was faced with a deficit of £17000. This was mainly due to a fall in voluntary subscriptions and when, in the following year, he launched an appeal for £200000 to maintain the hospital for the next five, he can hardly have been optimistic. The slump continued, unemployment remained widespread, the cost of living high. In spite of superhuman efforts the quinquennial appeal of 1933 raised only £80000. Two years later he was forced to appeal to the public again. 'During my chairmanship,' he wrote to *The Times* in desperation, 'the income of the Hospital has just met the ordinary expenditure, but it has not enabled us to reduce our heavy load of debt. It is for the means to enable the Hospital to maintain its position that I now appeal.' Again his appeal was only partially successful and in his report for the year he was compelled to tell the governors that it was 'becoming increasingly difficult to make provision for capital improvement of any kind'.

He was certainly in an unenviable position. On one side he had to face the British people, sick to death of hospital and other charitable appeals and, in general, ignorant of the rising cost of medical treatment; on the other, his own professional staff who were for ever (as it must have seemed to him) demanding some new department or the purchase of some expensive equipment and, unrepresented on the house committee, in general ignorant of the desperate financial straits into which the hospital had sunk. He also had to decide between their repeated claims and the urgent necessity of finding better accommodation for domestic and nursing staff.

To add to his troubles the cost of medical practice rose as new discoveries came along. The introduction of liver extract in the treatment of pernicious anaemia followed hard on the discovery of insulin, and that could cost up to a pound a day per patient. Radium had been given to the hospital by the Medical Research Council from which radon was now prepared and used in the treatment of malignant disease. A radon laboratory with expert staff had become a necessity. X-rays, too, were now employed in treatment, and bigger and better apparatus seemed to him to be in almost continuous demand. X-ray diagnosis was also being rapidly extended. Not only were bones X-rayed, but the chest was as well, and the technique of filling cavities such as the stomach with opaque barium was being rapidly extended. The bill for X-ray films had soared; the equipment in the department of X-ray diagnosis now lagged far behind that which the medical staff maintained was their right to expect!

Specialization both in medicine and surgery was also well under way, demanding capital outlay and increasing maintenance costs at each successive step. Surgeons were beginning to operate on the chest, as cancer of the lung became increasingly common, and Tudor Edwards was invited from the Westminster to 'the London' to start a department of thoracic surgery. Henry Souttar, that versatile genius who had been the first to operate on the mitral valve of the heart, was now experimenting in the surgery of the brain and inspired his house surgeon, Hugh Cairns (a Rhodes scholar who joined the college soon after the war); he was beginning to take a serious interest in nuero-surgery. Cairns went to the USA, studied under Harvey Cushing and, on his return, was appointed in charge of a neuro-surgical unit of his own. A man of strong physique (he had rowed in the Oxford boat) and incredible energy, dedicated to his work, he must be regarded, with Geoffrey Jepherson of Manchester, as one of the two pioneers of neuro-surgery in this country.

In addition to the medical unit, financed by the university, a Freedom Research Fund of £50000 had been established by an anonymous donor and important work was now in progress in hospital and college: on the metabolism of bacteria; on the radiology of the heart; on protein structure; on the chemistry of immunity; on stapyllococcal antitoxin. Howard Florey was working on body fluids (he returned to Oxford before he started to exploit Fleming's discovery of penicillin). Bedson, who had succeeded Bullock as professor of bacteriology, had become the leading authority on virus disease and, when a number of cases of psittacosis (parrot disease) were admitted to the hospital, succeeded in establishing its virus nature. A born teacher, he was a pillar of support to the medical college. In the dental school, Harold Chapman had become a leading authority on orthodontics. Evelyn Sprawson had been appointed dental surgeon to Dr Barnardo's Homes. 'It was in connection with these children,' writes Professor Miles, 'that he made one of the first studies of dental decay under controlled environmental conditions which resulted in a publication important, not only as to its conclusions, but also as a demonstration of method.'

In the field of morbid anatomy, Turnbull's reputation was now international. In Germany post-vaccinial encephalomyelitis was known as Turnbull's disease! He had also shown that high blood pressure comes first; that arterial degeneration follows after. 'The Chief was a scholarly man,' writes Donald Hunter, 'and did a great deal to foster accurate work in others. Above all he was modest, fully recognizing that humility is the prerequisite of all learning. The natural bent of his mind was academic and he exhibited that disinterested intellectual curiosity which has been called the life blood of real civilization. Ignorance he would condone but he never conceded his distaste for slipshod thinking, and he tried to inculcate in us habits of exact and accurate observation, orderly and relevant arrangement of thought, and critical judgement. These attainments he carried with natural ease himself. As has been said of John Hunter his greatness was revealed, not so much as a discoverer of new entities, but by his example in the use of the scientific method, in purity of heart and with utter devotion to truth. Turnbull had a quality which was distinctly spiritual. It inspired his pupils. We felt the urge of a great leader and we did his bidding, not out of fear, but out of respect and devotion.'

In 1935 the King celebrated the 25th anniversary of his accession. Even the mean streets of Whitechapel were decorated and for 'the London' it was a great occasion. For, in a recent attack of pneumonia, complicated by empyema (suppuration in the pleural cavity), he had been nursed at the Palace by London Hospital nurses like his father before him, and looked after by London Hospital doctors. Now, within a year of his Jubilee, he was again taken ill. Again he was nursed by London Hospital nurses, and it was Lord Dawson, his physician, who in January 1936 announced to the waiting world that the King's life was 'moving peacefully to its close'.

Meanwhile, the brief spell of optimism associated with the Jubilee and engendered by the gradual passing of the trade depression and decrease in unemployment, largely due to re-armament, had faded. The international scene had darkened; vague hope in the possibility of peace was fast giving way to a dull acceptance of the inevitability of war. In the hospital, Professor Wright had died, and I had been appointed dean. In a sense the world now seemed at my feet, the school flourishing, but the international scene continued menacing, and the hospital, on which the school depended, was daily sinking deeper into debt.

Subscriptions had been falling off for some time and now this thin stream of charity was drying up in favour of refugees abroad. An appeal to the public had to be made if the hospital was to keep up to date, let alone survive. As the next quinquennial appeal fell due in 1938 and the hospital would be celebrating its bicentenary in 1940, the governors decided to launch an appeal extending over three years in which they would ask for £270000 for capital development and £60000 to meet the increasing cost of maintenance. A brochure explaining the needs of the hospital was published, and the Lord Mayor agreed to a banquet at the Mansion House in May, at which the Duke of Kent consented to preside. At this the great appeal to the public would be officially launched.

Three months before the day the international situation deteriorated still further. Hitler forcibly incorporated Austria into the Reich and soon after started to stir up trouble in Czecho-slovakia. Early in May 1938 reports of German troop movements raised fears of a sudden attack. But Hitler held back and no immediate crisis followed. So the banquet at the Mansion House was held as planned in spite of the now tense international situation, the Archbishop of Canterbury and Lord McMillan appealing eloquently on the hospital's behalf, stressing the needs of the hospital or, as it was called at its foundation, 'the Charity'.

June, July and August proved months of suspense. In Czechoslovakia, Lord Runciman was endeavouring to settle the Sudeten question. In this country, rearmament was accelerated and civil defence was in the slow process of its tardy birth, but nothing had yet been decided by the ministry as to what should be done about air-raid casualties in the event of war. In the hospital, the main preoccupation at the moment, trivial though that may seem looking back now in relation to coming events, was finding a new matron to replace Miss Littleboy, an 'old Londoner' of the Lückes school who had done her job well within her limitations. This time the medical staff was determined to have an 'old Londoner' who had also gained experience elsewhere, and the house committee eventually agreed to the appointment of Miss Mabel Reynolds, matron of the London Clinic in Harley Street. Her attitude to life was certainly more liberal than that of any of her predecessors. She had also backed the movement, now gaining strength, for the better technical training of nurses. Qualified sister tutors were appointed; under her matronship, the one-time probationer became the student nurse.

In mid-September the European situation came to a sudden head. Hitler appeared to be on the verge of attacking Czechoslovakia but agreed to meet Chamberlain at Berchtesgaden. Then, at Godesberg, with French approval, agreement was reached on the orderly cession to Germany of all districts in the Sudetenland with a population more than half German. When, however, Chamberlain returned to Germany, Hitler demanded the immediate cession of all the German-speaking areas. Chamberlain refused. On the night of Tuesday, 27 July, war with Germany seemed certain.

A state of emergency was declared. Gas masks were issued to civilians, basements, underground stations, warehouses and cellars hurriedly converted into public shelters. Navvies started digging trenches in the parks. Plans were made for the evacuation of children from large cities. 'The London' received instructions to stand by to evacuate patients at twelve hours' notice and get ready to take in air-raid casualties, but no one seemed to know where the former were to be sent. No plans yet seemed ready for the deployment of nursing and medical personnel in the event of war.

The hospital, too, like every other institution of its kind, was completely unprepared for air attack. Lay, medical and nursing staff now got busy in their respective spheres to meet it. Fire was the major risk, and the house governor and surveyor organized students and porters into fire-fighting squads and they, in the meanwhile, filled and piled up sandbags to protect doors and windows. A committee, under the chairmanship of Russell Howard, senior surgeon, which included the matron and house governor (and of which, as physician and dean, I was a member) sat all day, attempting to reorganize the hospital to deal with air-raid casualties. These, we decided, should be sorted in the receiving room, special wards being set apart for gas and traumatic cases. The theatres on the top floor would be closed, and emergency ones fitted up in the basement. Blood transfusion teams were organized; students detailed as dressers and stretcher bearers, and certain members of the staff for special duties. In general the staff, both medical and nursing, carried on their normal work in complete ignorance of what would happen to them, or of what they might suddenly be called upon to do, if war came. What would have happened if Hitler had launched an air attack on London at that time, and it had got through, defies all imagination.

Uncertainty reigned supreme. Then the unexpected Munich settlement led to a sudden temporary release of tension. But 'Peace with honour' was soon called in question and the hope of 'peace in our time' did not last long. It was now abundantly clear that detailed plans, which would operate automatically in the event of war, must be made quickly. Never must the country be caught unprepared, as it had so nearly been.

The problem of air-raid casualties had begun to cause great public anxiety. The forecast was truly horrific. Over 3000 tons of high explosive, it was calculated, might be dropped on central

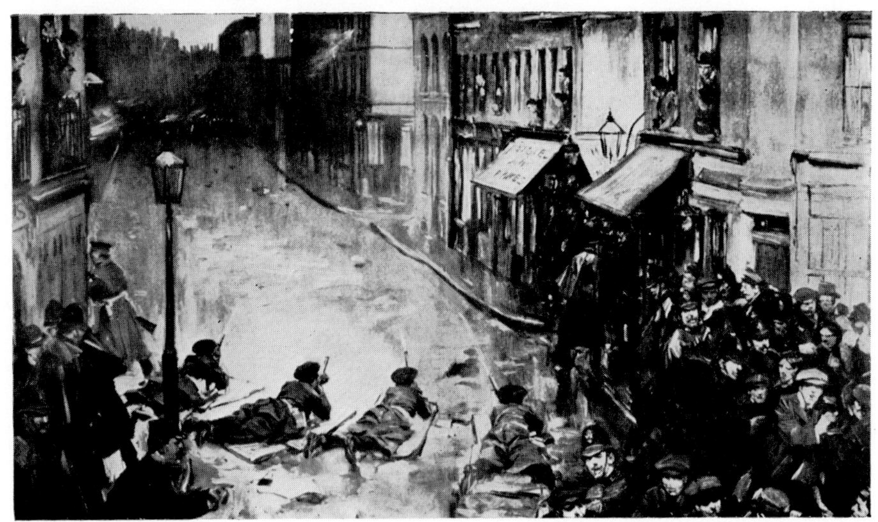

THE BATTLE OF SIDNEY STREET

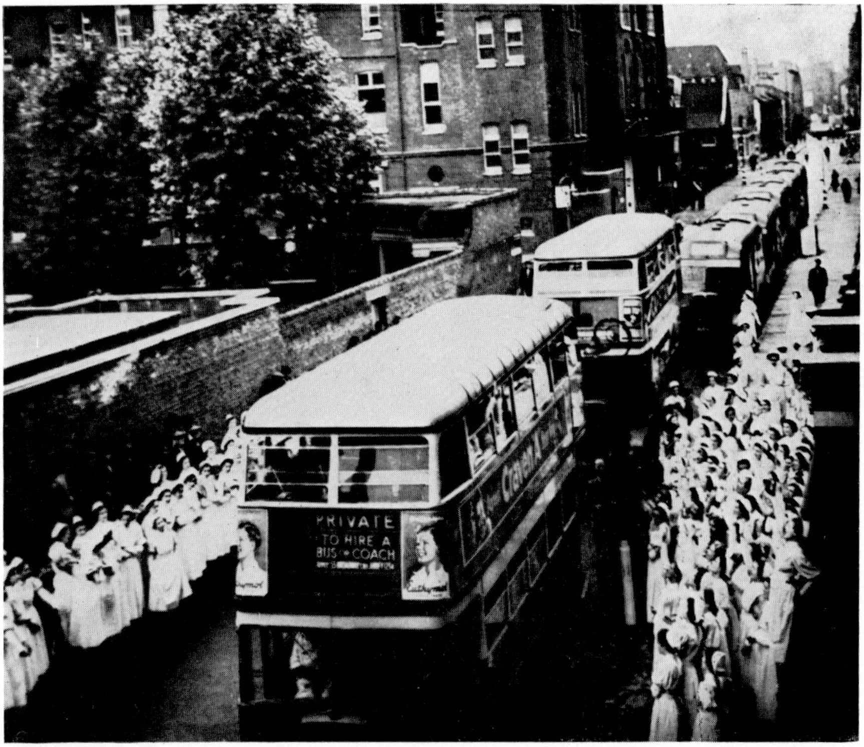

THE EVACUATION OF PATIENTS AND NURSES TO THE COUNTRY ON
2ND SEPTEMBER 1939

THE GERMAN AIR-RAID ON THE DOCKS ON 7TH SEPTEMBER 1940

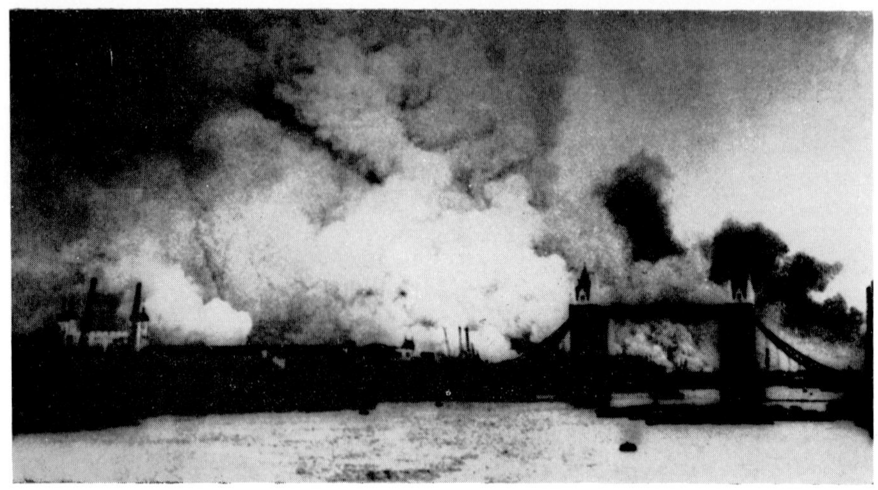

BICENTENARY DAY
Laundry workers greet the King and Queen with the Chairman, Sir William Goschen

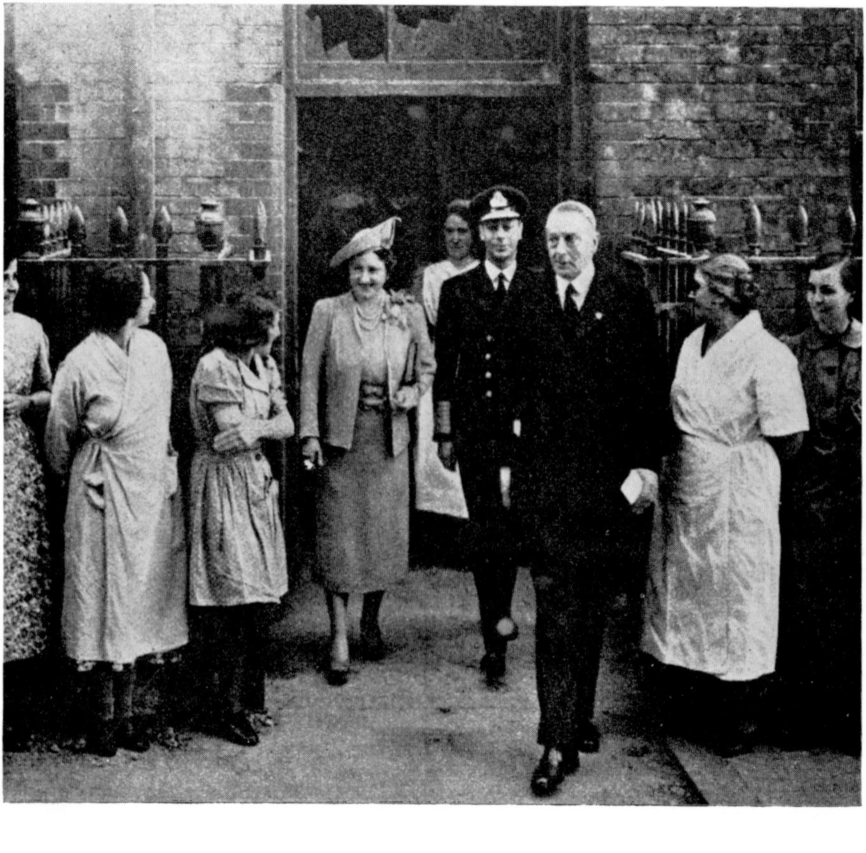

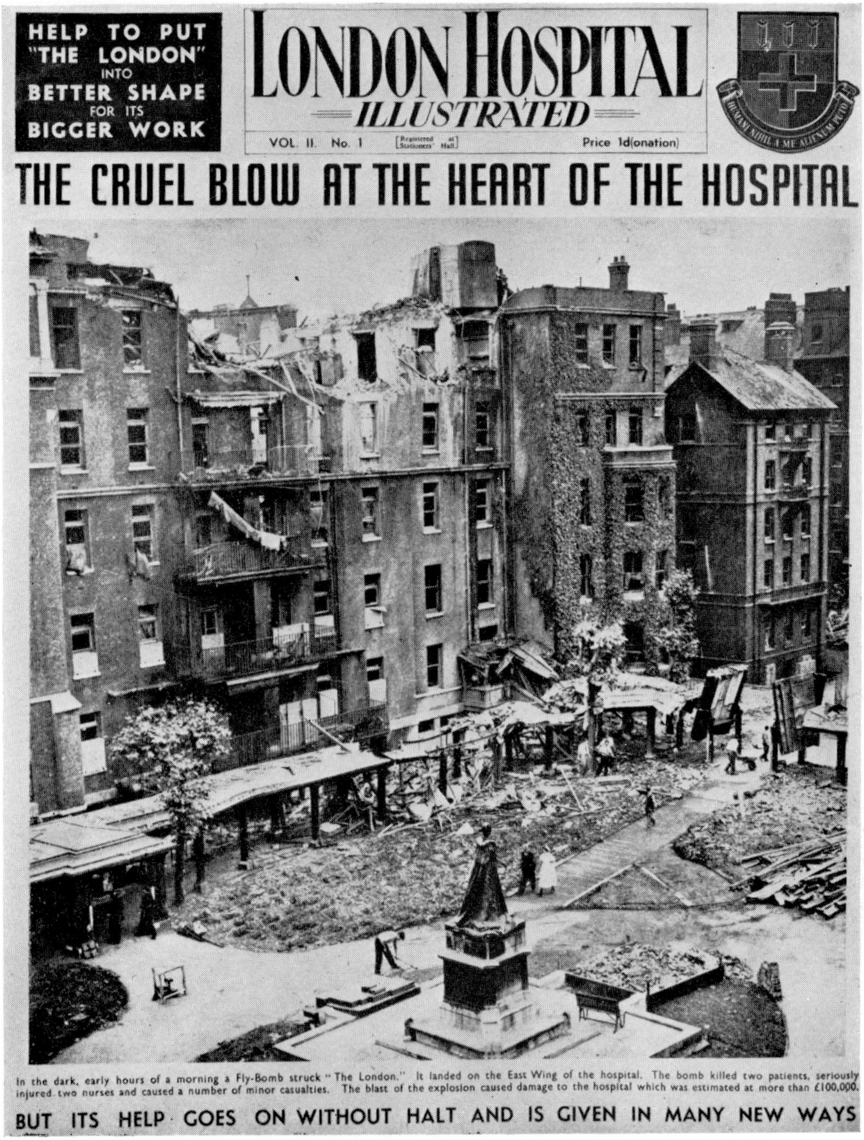
HELP TO PUT "THE LONDON" INTO BETTER SHAPE FOR ITS BIGGER WORK

LONDON HOSPITAL ILLUSTRATED

VOL. II. No. 1 [Registered at Stationers' Hall] Price 1d(onation)

THE CRUEL BLOW AT THE HEART OF THE HOSPITAL

In the dark, early hours of a morning a Fly-Bomb struck "The London." It landed on the East Wing of the hospital. The bomb killed two patients, seriously injured two nurses and caused a number of minor casualties. The blast of the explosion caused damage to the hospital which was estimated at more than £100,000.

BUT ITS HELP GOES ON WITHOUT HALT AND IS GIVEN IN MANY NEW WAYS

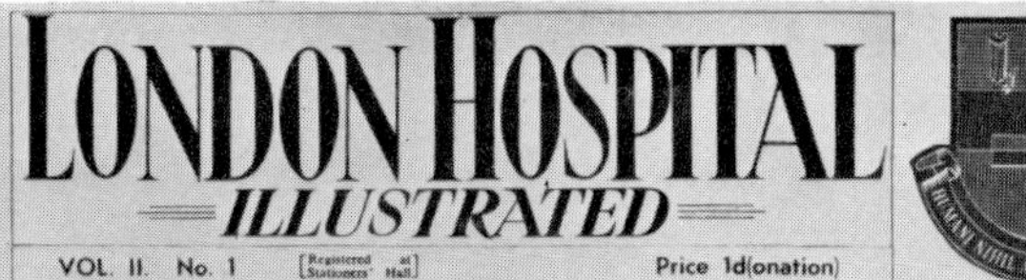

WHEN DAYLIGHT CAME ON 3RD AUGUST 1944

The East Wing wrecked by a flying bomb

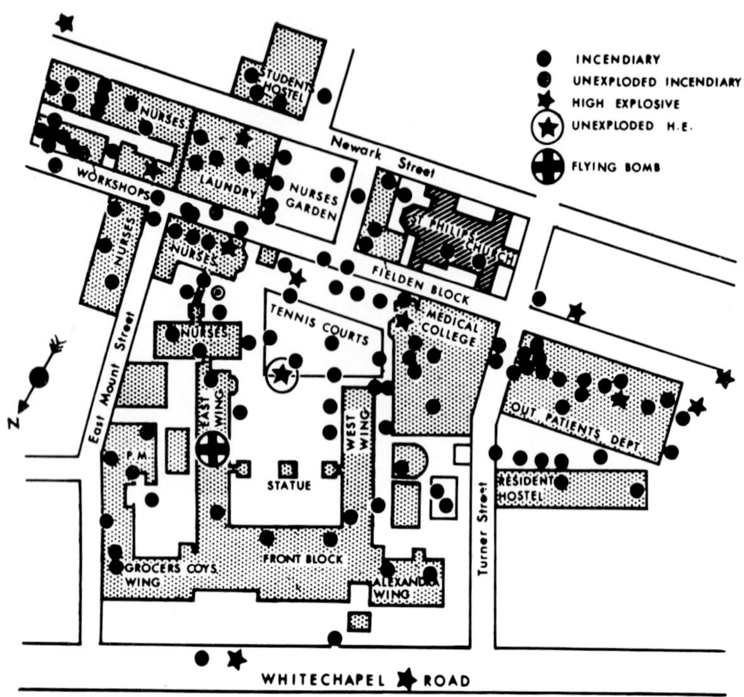

WHERE EACH BOMB FELL

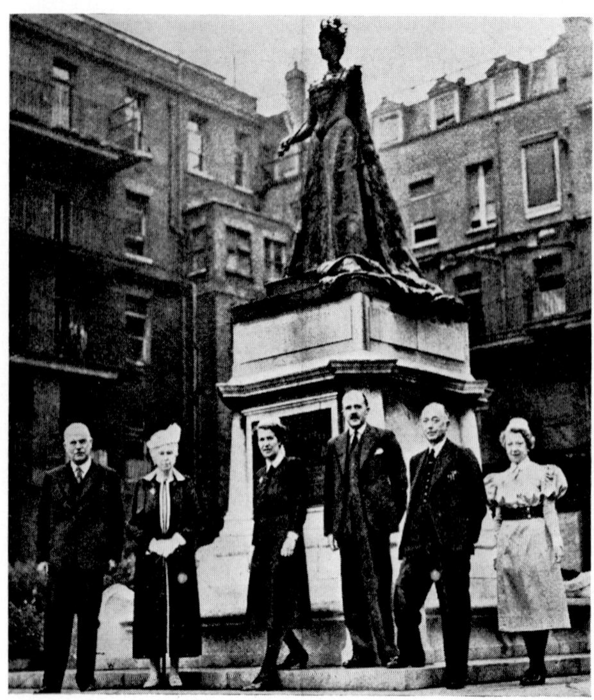

ONE OF QUEEN MARY'S MANY VISITS
Left to right: Sir John Mann, Queen Mary, Miss Alexander, Capt. Brierley, George Neligan, Miss Walker

London in the first twenty-four hours of a war; up to 400000 casualties, it was thought, could be expected. So the ministry decided, in the event of war, to reduce the staff of all the hospitals in central London to skeleton proportions and transfer all staff thus rendered redundant, and as much essential equipment as possible, to those outside London, many of these, particularly those in evacuation areas, to be enlarged by building huts and others to be upgraded, as the ministry put it, to undertake work of a kind to which they were entirely unaccustomed.

This scheme entailed both the transfer of equipment and er-deployment of the medical and nursing personnel, so London and the surrounding country were divided into ten administrative sectors radiating from Charing Cross. In each of these a senior consultant was now appointed as group officer to advise the ministry on the coordination of the work of all the voluntary and municipal hospitals in the area, and on the recruitment of the honorary staff of the voluntary hospitals in it into a salaried Emergency Medical Service. Although these group officers had no executive authority, their appointment did much to relieve the growing anxiety of the public as to the apparent com-placency of the government as to air-raid casualties in the event of war.

Sectors I and II were allotted to 'the London'. They included east and north-east London, the whole of Essex and parts of Middlesex and Hertfordshire. Russell Howard was appointed group officer. Something of a rough diamond, a typical 'Lon-doner' of his generation, forthright and full of common sense, he was universally trusted, but he had no previous experience of administration and possessed little flair for it. So, at his request, I was appointed to assist him. My job was to act as his adjutant, keep him organized, and rescue the daily bundle of unanswered letters which protruded from his pocket!

We were presented with a list of the hospitals in our area which would provide EMS beds for air-raid casualties and sickness among evacuees and to which, in the event of war, we would direct surplus staff and to which I would allocate students to act as dressers and continue their medical education. For, if war came, medical students all being 'reserved' this time, I would need to maintain a decentralized medical school as best I could. This list revealed a mixed lot, the hospitals in it falling into three main categories. First, there were the LCC hospitals in east and north-east London, the one time poor-law infirmaries. These would have to be handled with tact, being suspicious of voluntary hospital interference. This group also included two large fever hospitals which would provide a large reserve of beds for air-raid casualties, if the need arose. Secondly, there were the other voluntary hospitals in our area. They presented no particular problem and would clearly be useful to me as dean in trying to keep the medical school alive. They would carry on their work, we imagined, more or less as usual, even in a war. Thirdly, there were the county general and county mental hospitals in Essex and Hertfordshire. These, we were told, were to be upgraded to deal with casualties and evacuees and that, although we might give advice, was clearly not our job. Our job was to redeploy medical personnel. Here we had a free hand. All our recommendations, those of the sector matrons (both 'Londoners'), and those of the house governor as lay sector officer responsible for the transfer of equipment and lay staff, were accepted without question by the ministry. The ministry, too, would provide all necessary transport and it would pay hospitals for EMS beds and for other services rendered by them, and also the salaries of doctors in the EMS, according to the nature of their appointments, when it came into being.

Were we getting ready for something so disastrous that it could never happen? Or, as the saying was then, would the balloon really go up one day? That was the state of mind prevailing throughout the early months of 1939. In high quarters optimism prevailed for a surprisingly long time. As late as the 15th of that fateful March Chamberlain referred to an impending era of tranquillity. In the same week *Punch* came out with a cartoon depicting John Bull as a civil defence warden, wearing a gas mask, and waking up from a bad dream, depicted as the spectre of war escaping out of the window! Then, on the very day that Chamberlain spoke, Hitler struck. German troops occupied Prague and a few days later England and France promised to support Poland if attacked. Mussolini invaded Albania and on 6 May the Rome–Berlin axis was converted into a military alliance.

War now seemed inevitable. Loading Green Line buses, which had been converted into ambulances for casualties, was rehearsed again and again. In the hospital it was feared that the wooden beams of Mainwaring's eighteenth-century building would hardly take the strain of any considerable fall of masonry. So Norman Oatley, the surveyor, started to shore them up with steel struts on every floor. Windows were protected with wire mesh within and borrowed lights covered with cellophane to reduce the risk of flying glass. Blacking out, to confrom with the regulations which would be enforced, proved time-consuming, expensive and difficult. There was no nice issue of suitable material by the government. Quantities of it, too, were required to render the hospital invisible at night. So London was scoured to find anything that might serve while sisters, nursing and domestic staff spent their spare time sewing curtains. Even when the job seemed nearly done, some windows still failed to satisfy the regulations and the candle power of the lights in many rooms and corridors would have to be reduced.

The risk of fire caused great anxiety. As roads and streets might well be blocked, the hospital would need to be completely self-supporting in respect of fire-fighting. Petrol trailer pumps were bought and porters and surveyors staff trained in their use. If the main water supply to the hospital failed, as fail it might, there were 70000 gallons in the nurses' swimming bath. (The donor had not thought in terms of that use for it when he so generously presented it!) Mains electricity would be almost bound to fail, so the theatres were provided with emergency lighting and a petrol engine installed in the basement to drive a dynamo to light all wards likely to be in actual use. Bunks were fitted up in the basements of the Fielden block, nurses' homes and college, and in the subway corridors of the hospital. Students started filling sand-bags to protect doors and windows, as at Munich, until blast walls could be built. No sand was available and earth had to be used instead. When spring came they sprouted and, as it turned out, most had begun to disintegrate by the time they were really needed.

The summer passed uneasily. 'In the event of war,' I said in my address at the prize-giving in the college that June, 'those who serve "the London" will be in a position of great responsibility. If, however, the peace of Europe can be maintained, our time will not have been wasted. The national effort of these days must inevitably leave a mark on the permanent structure of the country, and I believe that in making preparations for war, we are laying the foundation of a more efficient system in peace. One day some scheme will be evolved which will provide a hospital service for all sorts and conditions of men, and at the same time afford wider scope for medical education and an extended field for medical research. The work which we are doing now may well be the beginning of an organization which will ultimately combine the efficiency of municipal medicine with the long tradition of the voluntary hospitals for progress and service, a tradition firmly established in this place down the two centuries of our history.'

18

Into Battle

The holiday season came round again but few in a position of any responsibility dared to go away. Britain and France were endeavouring to persuade Russia to join in the guarantee of Poland. Hitler was negotiating secretly with Stalin, and suddenly 'the sinister news' of their non-aggression pact burst on the world like an explosion. A few days later Hitler unleashed his long premeditated attack on Poland.

Mussolini now intervened in a last-minute bid to keep the peace. He suggested a general conference to which Chamberlain agreed, provided Hitler withdrew his troops from Poland. So, for two days, the country waited in suspense while preparations for war were hurried hard ahead. Evacuation from danger areas began and children trooped away carrying their gas masks. In the hospital the surveyor worked all out to complete his shoring up of ceilings; the house governor worked round the clock transferring surgical equipment to sector hospitals, Turnbull's specimens to a cave at Godstone, and hospital radium to a clay pit in Bedfordshire. Operating theatres were improvised on the ground floor. Patients who could not be moved were collected there. Wards at the top of the building were closed, and the lower ones got ready for casualties, the total bed establishment of the hospital being reduced to 180 with 200 in reserve. Four hundred nurses with radiographers, dispensers, technicians and secretaries followed patients, not well enough to be sent home, to sector hospitals. Six senior members of the staff remained to hold the fort. The rest left, some to take up their prior commitments to the armed forces, the majority to embark on their appointments at the particular hospitals to which they had been allocated by the group officer. The medical college was closed, the contents of the museum stored in the basement, and, as I had arranged with the university, the junior, i.e. pre-clinical, students dispatched to Cambridge. Then I assembled the seniors in the lecture theatre and gave them their marching orders. A certain number were to stay behind to act as dressers. The rest I detailed in that capacity to thirty different widely scattered hospitals, promising that I would move them round from time to time and endeavour to keep the school alive and maintain their education as far as the unforeseeable future would permit. Then, as they gathered up their things and went their ways, I could not help wondering when or if I would see them all again.

At 11 a.m. on 3 September, as no reply to Mussolini's peace move had been received, Britain and France were at war with Germany again. The Prime Minister broadcast to the nation. Hardly were his words out of his mouth – 'it is evil things that we shall be fighting against and against them I am certain that right will ultimately prevail' – before the sirens wailed the first air-raid warning of the war. It was a false alarm. Further anticlimax now followed. No air raids came. No bombs dropped. The measures which had been so hurriedly adopted at the hospital to meet the expected emergency soon had to be modified. Within two days the out-patients department was reopened on a limited scale. Some hospital equipment was brought back. The resident staff started teaching. Discussions on all sorts of wide topics were held to while away the time. The lay staff organized a concert, the students a dance. 'So, you see, we have won the war of nerves,' wrote one of the latter, 'which, in our case, meant the war against boredom.'

Boredom was indeed the bogey which all and sundry now had to face. There was no war on land or in the air, and little on the sea, and, misled by the unexpected quiet and confronted with the difficulties of billeting, the tide of evacuees turned and started to flow back into London. So the war-time organization of the hospital soon had to be modified still further. The out-patients department was opened on a larger scale, and an almost normal service was maintained by the end of the year. Casualty beds were reduced to 160 and beds for ordinary cases increased to 300. Beds for private patients were even opened on the top floor of the Fielden block which, with the decline of sepsis and of the in-patient treatment of syphilis, had recently been adapted for that purpose.

Many of the medical staff found work at the hospitals to which they had been transferred, particularly those at the upgraded public assistance institutions where, out of the stream of medical progress, many of the inmates had never benefited from modern methods of treatment. At the upgraded mental hospitals, on the other hand, time hung heavy. Most of the London Hospital staff at them now opted for part-time work in the EMS, returned to private practice, and resumed their rounds at 'the London' as the wards filled up again. I resigned my appointment as assistant group officer. I returned to the hospital but spent much of my time driving round trying to maintain some semblance of organized medical education in my now far-flung medical school.

On the financial side there was less anxiety than might have been expected. Taxation had increased with the war and voluntary subscriptions fallen off, but the consequences of that had been more than offset by the now much decreased cost of running the hospital and by money received from the ministry for services rendered to the EMS. The latter included payment for maintaining casualty beds and the salaries and board of all London Hospital lay staff now working at sector hospitals. The financial year ended with a credit balance of over £2000!

The war seemed to have hung fire. Perhaps peace would be patched up somehow and nothing much happen after all? Anyhow, everyone now seemed to be thinking in terms of a better Britain and for some better medical organization for the country after the war, if there was really going to be one, was over. There were many reasons for this strange and almost epidemic state of mind. Everyone had been suddenly jolted out of the normal routine of his existence. Voluntary and county council hospitals had got mixed up together. Staff and students had seen for themselves the neglected holes and corners of the medical organization of the country, particularly the problems of the aged and chronic sick with which the county council hospitals and public assistance institutions remained under a statutory obligation to deal and which the voluntary hospitals had so far successfully evaded. The EMS had been formed to cope with the emergency of war. Now there was no war. Should not a national health service be organized to deal with the hospital needs of the nation in time of peace? Nor did the fact that the bicentenary appeal was dead stop the staff making grandiose plans for rebuilding the whole hospital somewhere on the estate. Daydreams of this kind dominated the minds of many during the strange period of the phoney war.

The first three months of the new year passed quietly and pseudo-optimism of this peculiar kind persisted. Then came the rude awakening. On 10 April Hitler invaded Denmark and occupied Norway. A British expeditionary force had to be withdrawn. Chamberlain was forced out of office and all that Churchill had to offer was 'blood, toil, tears and sweat'. Hitler launched his attack through the Ardennes. Belgium surrendered. The British army, divided from the French, was evacuated from Dunkirk. On 17 June Paris surrendered. Then Pétain sued for a separate peace, leaving Britain to fight for freedom all alone.

Invasion of England demanded mastery of the air and on 17 July Goering launched the Luftwaffe against the Channel ports and the ground installations of the RAF. Then, on Saturday, 6 September, two hundred bombers attacked the docks in broad daylight and fires were soon raging all down the north bank from Tower Bridge. No bombs fell near the hospital but casualties were admitted. So much water, too, had been used for putting out the fires that the hydraulic lifts went out of action and all patients were carried down to the ground floor. Orders were issued to the effect that, if further casualties were admitted during the night, a corresponding number of patients must be evacuated.

Sunday's daylight passed quietly. Then at 8 p.m. 320 bombers and 600 fighters returned to the attack, not against the docks this time, but against London. The resident staff had just finished dinner when the sirens sounded. A few minutes later bombs started falling. Then a whizz and a crash, and all dived for cover under the tables. A bomb had fallen in the road just outside the hospital and casualties started streaming in. The raid continued all night. The Alexandra and Lückes nurses' homes were hit, but no one hurt, and a fire quickly extinguished. Water had got into the gas pipes and breakfast the next morning was cooked on a battery of primus stoves.

This, then, was Hitler's *blitzkreig* at long last and, in view of the now probable shape of things to come, all patients fit to travel were hurriedly evacuated, the first floor opened and casualty beds increased to 200. But no raid followed for some days. The Battle of Britain was being fought out and on 15 September the Luftwaffe suffered its final defeat. 'Never in the history of human conflict,' Churchill told the House, 'has so much been owed by so many to so few.'

Hitler's plan of invading England had been frustrated and he now determined to bring this troublesome island to its knees by the indiscriminate bombing of its large cities. London was raided almost every night at first. About an hour after sunset the sirens would sound and the inhabitants of Whitechapel soon learnt to seek refuge in the underground stations or deep shelters now provided by local authorities. Some old people started to live in them. Others refused to leave their homes. The drone of the coming planes would now be heard and then the crash of bombs and the rumble of falling masonry. At first these attacks seemed unopposed but, on the night of the 11th, the barrage opened with a roar – one big gun near the hospital shaking the building every time it fired – and circling searchlights lit the sky. Then, in the morning, came the aftermath of the night before: weary humanity trailing home from the undergrounds and shelters; figures searching for relatives and property among the ruins of their homes, the characteristic smell of the recently blitzed area; the soon familiar noise of the sweeping up of broken glass. Weariness prevailed at first. But before long the relentless regularity of these attacks had found its match in a dogged determination in East

London to stick it out, no matter what the cost. There was no panic in Whitechapel as in the First World War.

In the hospital everybody soon settled down to their routine. After dinner in the basement the staff picked up their tin hats and proceeded to their allotted posts: the house governor and secretary to their office, whence one of them always toured the wards when a raid was on; the surveyor to his control centre and his men to their observation stations to report where bombs fell or incendiaries landed; the doctors to the receiving room, resuscitation room and theatres. Where Turnbull went was uncertain but, bereft of company in the mess, as often as not he elected to continue his researches in his department despite the fact that there he was encased in unprotected glass. In the wards, sisters and nurses put on their tin hats and continued their work. Miss Burgess, the acting matron – matron had been transferred to sector headquarters – glided round the wards, leaving a trail of confidence and kindliness behind.

On 17 September the first land mine floated down on a parachute and devastated a large area just south-east of the hospital. Three days later a bomb fell between the out-patient building and the new department of physical medicine. Miss Burgess was knocked down and cut by flying glass. Three delayed-action bombs fell on the hospital estate. Another of the same type necessitated closing the out-patient department until the bomb disposal squad had dealt with it according to their art. Street after street would now be closed with the notice UXB. A bicycle, I soon found, was much the most practical way of getting about.

On our 200th anniversary day the King and Queen visited the hospital. That same evening, just after a rather better dinner than usual, there came a startling nearby whizz – but no explosion. We went out to investigate. A gaping hole had appeared in the garden where the statue of Queen Alexandra stands, caused presumably by a delayed-action bomb that might go off at any moment. Wards at risk were cleared as far away and as quickly as possible. But we had to wait six whole days – while this menace persisted – before Lieutenant Davies, who had defused the bomb that threatened St Paul's, came down with his team to deal with it.

Our bomb, for some technical reason, could not be defused. It had to be covered up with tons of earth and detonated. These tons now went up into the air. No windows had been broken, but tattered sandbags, caught up in the telephone wires crossing the garden, persisted drearily for weeks.

Early in October the Germans started dropping incendiaries. Fire-watching became a statutory duty. This was shared between the students and the surveyor's staff. Many fires were started but all quickly put out except one in the Lückes Home. This blazed for two hours before it was extinguished with water out of the swimming bath.

A week later, in the middle of dinner, a succession of whizzes and bangs swept across from the direction of Aldgate. All dived under the tables for cover again (I can remember hitting my head hard against that of the professor of medicine in the mêlée). The college had been hit; that was clear almost at once, and its sole occupant, my lame secretary (to whom I had given permission to sleep there during the week as she had difficulty in getting home at night), emerged shaken but unhurt from the basement. A bomb had fallen through the roof, exploded on the concrete floor of the dissecting room – empty even of dead bodies – and blown the bacteriology laboratory to pieces. The first of the stick had fallen in Aldgate, the second in the Whitechapel Road. It was the third which had hit the college. The fourth destroyed a tree in the garden, and the fifth had narrowly missed the students' hostel, built just before the war out of the subscriptions of 'old Londoner's' and a generous grant from the Knutsford memorial fund, in Ashfield Street.

The winter was now on us and the number of beds in action in the hospital for ordinary cases was increased to 350 to meet the higher rate of sickness expected. The Blitz itself was not associated with any increase in it. Rather, the reverse seems to have been the case, the population of London healthier than before to a degree difficult to account for in terms of orthodox medicine. Shelter life bred its diseases: gravitational oedema, bed sores, pressure palsies. But there was no appreciable increase in respiratory and gastro-intestinal infection as had been feared. Indeed, it is difficult not to conclude that the community spirit and that of mutual help engendered by hatred of a common enemy, and determination to stick it out, had raised resistance to disease above its average level.

Longer nights and shorter days favoured the raiders. Raids continued regularly until 3 November when there was a sudden almost sinister silence. Goering had switched his attack to the industrial cities in the north. London's respite was, however, brief. Ten days later the Luftwaffe returned to the attack and on 29 November, chosen deliberately because the tide in the river would be low, came the big raid on the city. That night the hospital was full of smoke. St Peter's in Vallance Road, a one-time infirmary very near the hospital, was badly damaged and its patients admitted to 'the London'. Additional wards had to be opened to cope with the situation.

Raids became less frequent (most nights, in fact, quiet) as our defences improved, the Germans lost more and more planes, and Goering concentrated his attack on other cities, notably Coventry, Birmingham, Bristol and Plymouth. As the raids diminished in number, however, they gained in intensity. Bombs got larger, incendiaries started to explode, land mines became more frequent. Oil bombs were also dropped. On 11 January many incendiaries fell on the roof and the hospital took in thirty of the casualties that resulted from the bomb which fell on the Bank. On 8 March bombing continued for five hours, many bombs falling in the neighbourhood. Again the lifts failed and, as the Bishopsgate telephone exchange was hit, the hospital was left out of all communication with the outside world. Three days later 'the London' suffered its greatest raid of incendiaries: thirty-four fell on it. All were extinguished before they had started fires of any magnitude.

On 11 March another raid on the docks started at 8.30 p.m. and continued until 4 a.m. A bomb on Whitechapel station, opposite the hospital, blew in windows, and a number fell just to the east of it. Seventy-six casualties were admitted, and a second resuscitation ward had to be opened. The London Chest Hospital in Victoria Park was damaged by a land mine, and four injured nurses were transferred to 'the London'. A month later, on 16 April, there was another heavy raid in the vicinity. Forty casualties were taken in, incendiaries fell all round and fire broke out in the carpenters' shop. Norman Oatley was slightly injured. Three days later came another bad night. Bombs fell just to the west of the hospital and St Peter's, the old infirmary in Vallance Road immediately north of it, was seriously damaged by a land mine and caught fire. The house governor went over and took charge. Its thirty-six patients were transferred to 'the London'.

On 10 May windows were blown in, doors dragged off their hinges, cupboards sucked open. The lifts went out of action again. All the essential services failed. Poplar was hit and patients from it evacuated to 'the London'. Mann's brewery just down the road was hit and twenty-five of their horses killed. The remainder galloped terror-stricken up the road to be deflected by our porters, who lined up across it, into the hospital car park. There they were tied up for the night.

This, although not realized at the time, was the last raid of the Blitz – Hitler was moving his bombers and fighters away to support his coming invasion of Russia – and looking back now it is clear that 'the London' had been incredibly lucky. Although it had been hit eight times by high explosives, although scores of incendiaries had rained down on it causing two serious fires, although devastation reigned all round, it had never been seriously damaged. Nor had a single doctor, nurse or member of the lay staff been seriously hurt. The number of casualties taken in was 1330, a surprisingly small number in view of the official estimates before the war.

No operation had been attempted on the seriously injured until a patient was declared sufficiently recovered from shock. Blood transfusion saved many lives. All casualties had been given tetanus antitoxin and sulphonamides to arrest infection. (Pencillin had still to be discovered.) Head injuries, chest wounds and injuries of the lower limbs had been allotted priority in respect of evacuation, the latter because, in the event of fire, they would have been difficult to move. For this we had been fully prepared. All beds had been provided with a rope fitted underneath the mattress. This could have been twisted over it and the patient pulled out of the ward and downstairs on the floor.

Three people throughout that testing time stand out in my
memory. George Neligan's experience as a surgeon in the First
World War had stood the hospital in good stead, but his personality had contributed something to the psychology of the
situation which was even more valuable. The life, it is true, suited
his unhurried Irish temperament. There he would sit hour after
hour, his cup of coffee or tankard of beer before him, smoking
cigarette after cigarette, his meditations only interrupted by fits of
coughing, an unparalleled example of imperturbability to all
who were privileged to work with him. Never have I come
across another man who managed to go through the motions of
doing so little and yet at the same time succeeded in accomplishing
so much. Conscious of everything that was going on, he was
always there when wanted; watching quietly to see that everything went right; never saying a word unless he saw that something wrong would be done if he did not intervene. Even then,
never did he claim the credit for a right decision.

On the house governor, Henry Brierley, the entire responsibility for the safety of the hospital had rested and as lay sector officer
it had been his duty to cope with every other hospital emergency
near by. Never did he falter, either. He inspired confidence everywhere and his capacity for quick and right decisions had proved
invaluable again and again. To the friendly disposition of the
surveyor must be attributed the efficiency of his staff. Again and
again, too, Norman Oatley's physical courage, and that of his
men, had saved the hospital from disaster. Nor can I ever forget
old Turnbull either. Exactly why he was there is not clear. To the
casualty service he contributed nothing but the spectacle of
academic work as usual in spite of the Blitz, was, to say the
east of it, inspiring. He seemed to us all, too, to constitute a
link between a world that had suddenly evaporated and one which,
all lived in hope, might one day come back again.

So ended this episode in which 'the London' had helped London
to take it. No claim is made that it did more than any other
hospital but let George (Neligan) pay *his* tribute to all who worked
with him. 'It is impossible to find words', he wrote, 'to express
one's appreciation of the behaviour of the whole staff whether

they were sisters, nurses, medical or lay. *They were a grand team who never faltered.* Going round the wards during a raid it was good to see the sisters and nurses working all out, the only noticeable difference from peace-time being their tin hats, often worn at jaunty angles, on their heads, in spite of the noise of the guns and falling bombs repeatedly shaking the building. Another section of the staff I shall never forget' – and here he had in mind all the humbler workers – 'were the old night scrubbers. Many of these were over seventy, and for untold years had turned up at 6 a.m. to clean the same area of hospital floor. Now, no matter how severe the blitz, or whether transport had been knocked out and they had to walk from their homes, many of which had been ruined by bombs, these old ladies turned up to time, and pail in hand would settle down to their long-accustomed task, only stopping to argue from time to time with their scrubber friends as to who had had the biggest bomb dropped near her during the night.'

19

Bombs and Rockets

There had now been no air raids for some time. Official opinion, however, remained pessimistic as to whether Russia would be able to withstand the German onslaught, and a quick German victory would certainly have led to renewed air attacks on Britain. The Blitz might then return; gas, possibly, might even still be used. The ministry would not allow any more beds to be opened in the hospitals in central London for the moment.

Meanwhile, the hospital continued to benefit financially, for it continued to be paid by the ministry for the EMS beds which it provided, and these continued to stand empty, costing next to nothing to maintain. So a peace-time deficit had now become a war-time surplus. During the first full year of the war the income of the hospital exceeded expenditure by over £40000!

The voluntary hospitals, the ministry therefore thought, should make some effort to establish country branches in order to help in the treatment of the ordinary sick. 'The London' now undertook to rent and run a hutted hospital adjacent to the LCC hospital for children at Brentwood in Essex. London Hospital patients would be admitted to it directly, nursed by London Hospital nurses and cared for by London Hospital staff. All the main branches of medicine and surgery were to be represented and, when it was opened, I was able to dispense with many of the sector hospitals, which I had hitherto been compelled to use for teaching, and transfer the students at them to our annexe at Brentwood.

The nursing had suffered even more than the medical school from dispersal at the beginning of the war and from the more recent chaos of the Blitz. Never had it been easy to maintain London Hospital standards or organize the training of London Hospital nurses in 'other people's' hospitals. The unity, too, of the nursing school had been disrupted by the war. Miss Reynolds had been matron of Sector I, and now shared responsibility for the training of London Hospital nurses with Miss Burgess, acting-matron at 'the London', and with Miss Walker, now matron of Sector II. The situation was, in fact, awkward and only resolved by the resignation of Miss Reynolds. This left the house committee free to act. Miss Alexander, an 'old Londoner', was now offered the matronship of 'the London' and accepted it on the understanding that she became matron of both sectors and ran them from 'the London', in this way gaining control of the nursing at all the hospitals where 'London' nurses were working. The new matron must have spent as much time travelling round her far-flung nursing school as I had done, and to some extent was still doing, in trying to keep my scattered medical school together.

The menace of the war was now mainly from the sea. The sinking of merchantmen had increased. Rationing was in force and the feeding of patients becoming more difficult. Italy had come into the war, and we had lost control of the Mediterranean. The Japanese had attacked the American fleet in Pearl Harbour without warning. To many people this seemed another disaster. Churchill saw it differently. The United States were now in the war up to the hilt which meant that we were bound to win in the end. Everything now merely depended on 'the proper application of overwhelming force'.

Britain had a long way to travel before the victory of which he was so confident would be achieved. For the moment, however, the German offensive against Russia, Japanese intervention, fighting in the Balkans and the threat of an Italian attack on Egypt conspired to keep the focus of hostilities well away from Britain. So, early in 1942, the ministry thought it safe to open more beds and allowed 'the London' to increase its complement

H

to 446 while still maintaining 336 at Brentwood. Many of the honorary staff out in the sectors now returned to work in the hospital or at Brentwood. Matron, too, brought back more nurses.

These changes were soon reflected in terms of total work done. In 1941, 6000 patients had been admitted to 'the London'. In 1942 this figure had risen to 8000 and out-patient attendance from 42000 to over 56000. Nor do these figures reveal all the work the hospital was doing. It continued to staff EMS hospitals at Chase Farm in Herts and Warley Woods in Essex; also to maintain two maternity homes, one in Essex and one in Herts. 'The London', although still scattered, was, as a matter of fact, almost twice as large as any other hospital at this time. It was doing more than twice their amount of work.

Other steps in reconstruction were also now considered safe. The school of physical medicine was brought back from Northampton; the radium and the radon laboratory from Bedfordshire. Certain innovations were permitted. Radiotherapy was separated from radiodiagnosis and a department of the former set up under the Cancer Act of 1939 to provide for East Anglia. A school of radiography was started, and an almoner's department to supplement the work of the Samaritan Society. Reginald Watson Jones was invited from Liverpool to get an orthopaedic and accident department under way.

Legacies, uninfluenced by the war, continued to fall in and during the first complete year of it reached a record of £103 740. One of them even ante-dated the Knutsford period; £62 393 from the estate of Mr Mercer, who had died in America in 1870, leaving a share of the residue of it to the hospital after the decease of certain beneficiaries. During 1941 legacies amounted to £59 000. In the following year the hospital was again lucky. Mr Fielden, who during his life had given the hospital over £84 000, had left it £100 000 in his will.

Acts of this kind led many to think that the voluntary system could still perhaps be saved. 'In the future the closest cooperation will be necessary,' wrote Sir William Goschen in his report to the governors, 'between the voluntary and the municipal hospitals in order to build up a hospital service for the country. The Government will continue to pay us for services rendered. *But there is no doubt in the minds of your Committee that it is in the best interests of the country that the voluntary system should be continued.*'

But could it continue? Was not the situation already too anomalous? The ministry was subsidizing the voluntary hospitals by paying them to maintain unoccupied EMS beds. The problem of the chronic sick remained. With the returning tide of evacuees the number of patients in this category had increased a hundred-fold and the municipal hospitals remained under a statutory obligation to them. The 'voluntaries' refused, as they had always refused, to block their beds with cases of this kind. So, while the municipal hospitals were now dangerously overcrowded, many of the 'voluntaries' remained relatively empty and their staff correspondingly underworked. It was, in fact, becoming increasingly clear that some unified hospital system for the whole country was needed. The dyarchy of voluntary and municipal hospitals must end. The middle of a great war, going badly for the country, was, however, hardly the moment to effect so radical a change.

The power of the Japanese military machine proved even greater than Churchill had expected. Singapore capitulated; the *Prince of Wales* and the *Repulse* were sunk. The loss of ships in the Atlantic increased. The Germans reinforced the Italians in North Africa and Rommel was hammering at the gates of Egypt. In June 1942 Tobruk surrendered and the 8th Army stood at bay.

In the hospital this was a depressing time. More of the honorary staff disappeared to join the services as the demand for specialists increased. The professor of medicine migrated to Oxford. We suffered losses, too, of other kinds. One of the anaesthetists was killed in an air raid. Russell Howard died. Sir William Goschen also died, in his own hospital like his predecessor. He had served it through hard times. He died when the future was beginning to look just a little brighter, just, in fact, as the tide of the war began to turn, for in the autumn of 1942 Montgomery defeated Rommel at Alamein. Alexander's victory of Tunis followed. The U-boat menace was got under control. Britain regained command of the

Mediterranean. In the following year Sicily was captured and the Allies landed in Italy. Plans were also already being concocted for the invasion of the Continent.

Fears were growing again, however, in the minds of those responsible for the defence of the U K. Rumours of Hitler's secret weapons had filtered through, and in May 1943 it became known that the Germans were experimenting with them in the Baltic. In August an attack by some form of pilotless aircraft seemed certain sooner or later, but the government now knew that, if need be, London could 'take it' and, although the hospitals were warned that large numbers of air-raid casualties were again to be expected, no plans were made for another evacuation. Reconstruction to meet demand was also allowed to proceed. By the end of the year 'the London' maintained 529 beds in Whitechapel and 345 at its annexe in Brentwood which, with seventy-five maternity beds in Hertfordshire, added up to 949. This was greater than the number maintained before the war. Out-patient attendances, too, now exceeded a thousand a day.

Permission was now gained to repair the Lückes Home to accommodate the increased number of nurses which the hospital required. Soon another hundred beds were opened. All the staff who had not joined one of the services came back, working primarily at 'the London' or Brentwood, or in both places, many still paying visits to their former sector hospitals as well. So I could now drop most of the latter as war-time teaching hospitals, and run the medical school almost entirely in Whitechapel and at Brentwood, maintaining only a skeleton service of students to act as dressers in other hospitals in central London in case of a renewal of the Blitz. Matron was able to recentralize her nursing school. London Hospital nurses were now withdrawn from all sector hospitals with the exception of Warley Woods and Chase Farm in order to serve 'the London' and the annexe at Brentwood. A second preliminary training school was opened. We were in fact, at least so it seemed at the time, fast returning to an almost normal way of life.

On 6 June 1944 the Allies launched their invasion of the Continent, taking the Germans, who had expected it much further

north, largely by surprise. This did not affect the hospital immediately – not till later did we start to take in casualties from
France – but shortly after this, as it happened, the Air Ministry
learnt that a number of railway waggons, carrying objects looking
like rockets, had passed through Ghent towards the Franco-
Belgian frontier.

One night a few days later I heard a plane flying low and, as it
seemed, uncertainly. Then its engine stopped and seconds later
came an explosion. It had crashed and blown up, I naturally
thought. Not so; it was one of Hitler's first pilotless aircraft which
had fallen at Bethnal Green, killing six people and injuring many
others. 'While I was Sister Gloucester,' writes Miss Mussared, 'I
had the first flying-bomb casualty, a woman with multiple
wounds and a severely mutilated arm. It took us 48 hours to get
her out of severe shock. Her chief concern then was for her
family. The almoner was able to trace the husband to a rest
centre and found that one boy had been killed, trying to save his
sister, and her other two children severely injured.'

An interlude of two days followed. Then these flying bombs
started coming at the rate of about a hundred a day. 'London now
has the privilege of sharing the dangers of the war with our forces
on the Continent', said Churchill, and in point of fact London
soon got used to them. Droning uncertainly across a few hundred
feet above the house tops they became almost a joke – doodle bugs
as some wag christened them – until the engine stopped. Then it
was time to take cover!

The Air Ministry redistributed their defences to meet this
attack. The anti-aircraft guns were redeployed and a cordon of
barrage balloons stationed between London and the coast;
fighters were ordered to chase and shoot these flying bombs
down. The former were soon accounting for 10 per cent, the
latter for 30 per cent. The rest got through and we had a grand
view of them coming over from the windows of the residents'
mess, now back on the first floor. On one occasion the engine
stopped, it seemed, just overhead. We all stopped eating. Then
crash – it had fallen on the bottling department of Mann's
brewery just down the road.

Before long everyone had begun to feel that our turn must come soon. It came in the early hours of the morning of 3 August. Matron was still working in her office. Norman Oatley had gone to bed but, having been wakened by an explosion not far away, was sitting on the edge of it convinced that the next one would be ours. Miss Gray, fed up with her bunk in the basement, had reverted to her own room and was sound asleep with her uniform draped over a chair, each garment in order ready to put on and her cap on top of them. I was asleep in my room in the residents' hostel to be wakened by the characteristic noise of an approaching bomb. Oldershaw, a student at the time, was fire-watching on the roof. 'We knew it was coming,' he writes. 'Many had gone over. One had just landed nearby and, simultaneously with its explosion, we heard the engine of another almost on top of us and the "imminent danger" warning of the klaxons. Then I saw it! It fell out of the low clouds, and I watched it diving for the Hospital, heard the final roar and sound of walls falling, shouting in the streets, doors opening and banging, all merged into seeing the building blazing with light through a cloud of rising dust.'

Sister Gloucester, who had been lying awake in a room on the ground floor, dived under her bedclothes. 'Plaster, broken glass and the cupboard doors showered on my bed, all lights went out, and my door jammed.' The house governor, who was in his flat on the ground floor of the Alexandra Home and also still awake, had heard the bomb coming, the engine stop, and then the swish of it descending. A crash followed. The ceiling came down and his wardrobe fell on top of him. The lights went off. He couldn't find his torch and so spent the next few desperate moments hunting for his trousers and his little Yorkshire terrier, which had been sleeping on his bed, in total darkness.

'At 1.35 a.m. I was sitting at the table in the middle of the ward,' night nurse Royal reported to matron. 'Everything was quiet; all the patients asleep. Suddenly I heard the sound of a flying bomb. The engine stopped and then I heard it whistling through the air and realized that it could hardly avoid hitting us. A moment later there was a terrific explosion, complete darkness, the crash of falling masonry, and the rush of water. Complete silence followed, and for a moment I feared that all my patients had been killed. So I began to grope my way in the darkness towards the lobby to fetch the hurricane lamp, but a soldier struck a match and I saw my torch lying on the table, switched it on, and he exclaimed, "Oh! nurse, you had better sit down" (I was bleeding from various cuts and scratches on my face and arm). I went to the patients near me and asked if they were all right. All answered cheerfully. Then, leaving the torch, I took the matches and went to the lobby for the hurricane lamp where I met Miss Burgess. I told her that I had lost my spectacles. She came back with me, and we went to the far end of the ward to see if the rest of the patients were all right. There we discovered a huge crater, and realized that the bed, containing a soldier, had completely disappeared.'

'Immediately the Hospital was in an uproar,' continues Older-shaw. 'Memories are incidental and fragmentary; two neat sisters in the receiving room; a house-man's white and preoccupied face; a nurse with no cap and her face and apron covered with dust; Civil Defence workers and soldiers pouring into the front hall. Captain Brierley, standing there with his hair on end, restoring order.' For everyone rapidly started to converge on 'the scene of the incident'. On his way across the garden he had found two nurses lying injured and mobilized stretcher parties to bring them in. (They had also been spotted by the fire-watchers on the Fielden block.) Bombs were now coming over in quick succession and matron ordered the children on the second floor, and all patients in immediate danger, to be moved down to the basement. George Neligan was quickly in the operating theatre to deal with the injured nurses (both of them subsequently recovered). Norman Oatley, having sized up the situation, rushed to the roof to try to stop the flood descending from above.

Orders were issued for the nurses to stay in their rooms; sisters to come on duty. Miss Gray's door was jammed but a colleague forced it open and she ran across the garden. 'A friend on the other side of the corridor', writes Miss Mussared, 'got my door open and with her help I got out, emptied my shoes of glass, and with the aid of her torch snatched up my uniform and dressed in the corridor. I made my way across the quadrangle which was piled high with broken masonry and rubble. I found the patients in Gloucester quiet and calm. In the lobby, water was cascading down from the roof and a fireman asked me for a dose of Broadbent's, in case he caught a cold!'

Quickly the ARP services arrived. Slowly the pattern of what had happened emerged. The bomb had fallen on the kitchen on the fourth floor and descended through the lobbies between the wards – had it done otherwise the casualty list would have been very different – blowing out the walls and floors of the wards on the second and third floors, which were empty. The heavy kitchen equipment had crashed down through the lobbies between the first and ground floors into the basement, opening up a vast crater over which one of the water storage tanks in the roof now hung suspended.

Gradually the situation was got under control by rescue squads assisted by the surveyor's staff, doctors and students, all heavily handicapped by the flood of water that continued descending from above. Further, a little later, a flying bomb hit Stepney Power Station, plunging the whole hospital into darkness until our own emergency lighting came on. A roll call now revealed that two patients were missing, presumably buried in their beds under tons of masonry and rubble, but, although everyone was white with dust, not a nurse or another patient had been hurt. The old Nurses' Home, the temporary X-ray hut and the covered way in the garden, which was littered with debris, had been badly damaged. Almost all windows in the hospital had been blown in, many doors dragged off their hinges, many cupboard doors wrenched off. All the blackout had been wrecked, and the hospital now stood out like a lighthouse in the darkness.

When daylight came all patients, other than those too ill to be moved, were transferred, with the nurses who knew them, to the annexe, Warley Woods and Chase Farm. The maternity patients were sent to Hitchin; the children, by arrangement with the ministry, to the Royal Northern Hospital. The medical college and the doctors' kitchens carried the extra load of work. A breakfast of eggs and bacon (a luxury almost unknown in wartime) was served at the usual time to staff, students and patients. 'While the damage to the Hospital has been heavy,' wrote the house governor in his report to the house committee, 'and there has been great loss of equipment and stores, the governors will be pleased to know that the Hospital never closed for the admission of patients, and by the evening there were 263 beds ready. There was no confusion of any kind, and I would like to pay a tribute to all the staff, medical, nursing, lay and domestic, who worked calmly and most efficiently through the early hours of 3rd August and the trying days since.'

Early in November a new menace was added to that of the flying bombs. Mysterious explosions, without any previous warning, started, first here, then there, puzzling everybody. The government was not entirely unprepared. During the previous months scraps of information had been collected which revealed that the Germans were experimenting with long-range rockets of about 12 tons weight, carrying a warhead of high explosive of round about a ton. Casualties on a large scale were now to be expected again and the hospitals had been warned accordingly; these rockets were to prove a very different proposition from Hitler's flying bombs. The latter could be shot down like birds, trapped in the balloon barrage like flies, and avoided when the engine stopped by taking cover. His rockets came too fast to be hit, and too high to be intercepted. No warning system was possible. So while the casualties from flying bombs remained low, those from these rockets proved to be much higher.

On 10 November one of the first to reach London fell in Petticoat Lane, the crowded market in East London. Over two hundred casualties were brought into the hospital and that night it was full to overflowing, extra beds having been put up in all the wards. A few days later, another fell in Aldgate. Again the receiving room was filled with stretcher cases and walking wounded, and four of the wards standing empty had to be opened. Students carried up mattresses and casualties were parked on the floor, irrespective of age and sex, waiting their surgical turn.

In December one of these rockets fell 100 yards from Warley Woods; on 5 January one fell in Stepney Way just behind the hospital; early in March another fell near the annexe in Brentwood; yet another fell in Commercial Road. Then at 7 a.m. on the 27th, a black cloud suddenly rose up just north of the hospital, followed a split second later by a roar. A rocket had fallen on a block of flats in long-suffering Vallance Road, killing 124 people. A few minutes later casualties on stretchers and walking wounded badly cut by flying glass crowded in through the main entrance of the hospital. Before long the mortuary was full, the dead lying outside, while a queue formed up seeking to identify relatives. Matron spoke to some of them and the mask-like face of a soldier who had returned from the front that morning to find his entire family destroyed remains imprinted on her memory.

Nine hours later Hitler's last rocket descended harmlessly in Kent. His launching sites were being liquidated as the war crescendoed to its close. By the beginning of April Eisenhower had crossed the Rhine. On the 25th Russians and Americans met on the Elbe. On 2 May Italy surrendered and Mussolini was shot by Communists. A few days later the German generals capitulated and Hitler took his own life. On 8 May the war in Europe had ended at long last.

Handing Over
to the State

Gradually members of the staff returned as demobilization of the armed forces gathered way – two from prisoner-of-war camps in Germany. They came back full of enthusiasm to start civilian life afresh, but found many changes awaiting them. The ruined east wing struck a desolate note. The damaged covered way in the garden added to the dreary scene. The number of beds had been severely cut, and many of the staff now had to endure the burden of driving all the way to the annexe to operate or resume their customary rounds.

Further, it soon became clear that the house governor, having been the man on the spot and run the hospital on his own for so long, held in his hands most of the power that the chairman and house committee had wielded before the war, and that an efficient matron, working hand in glove with him, as Miss Lückes had done with Lord Knutsford, had definite ideas of her own as to how the hospital should be organized. Not everybody liked this, and politics, largely disregarded for so long but ever at work in any vigorous self-governing institution, raised their head again. As in any healthy society, too, personalties began to clash. Henry Brierley, bred in the service tradition, had difficulty in understanding educational ideals which conflicted with his practical attitude to life. The concept of university freedom, too, ran counter to the need for discipline. On the other hand, he combined administrative efficiency with an amazing capacity for work, and all would agree that he had only one ambition: not the usual one of self-advancement, but the determination to further the reputation of 'the London' by every method which was, in his own opinion, likely to achieve that end. Here his singleness of purpose was remarkable. Maybe, he divided to rule, but never in its whole history has 'the London' possessed a more devoted servant.

The staff were coming back, too, at a time when medicine was advancing with extraordinary rapidity. Penicillin had been discovered in time for D-Day. Other antibiotics were being produced in quick succession. The treatment of tuberculosis had been revolutionized, and seventy beds already set apart for it at the annexe. Many discoveries in technology both in medicine and surgery, followed, in consequence of which physicians and surgeons began to specialize to varying degrees in one direction or another. Demands kept being made for new departments which, as I saw it, would cut across the organization of teaching and the normal pattern of medical education.

The house governor, primarily concerned with the treatment of patients and anxious to raise the reputation of the hospital, strongly favoured this movement, backed by many of the part-time members of the staff – that is to say, those also engaged in private practice. As dean, primarily concerned with the education of students, I felt, although in private practice myself, bound to oppose this trend and in so doing had the backing of the university members of the staff in full-time service of the hospital. Over-specialization was out of place, we both maintained, in an undergraduate school. Enough beds for general medicine and general surgery must be kept. It was impossible to teach medicine to students by putting them through a succession of special departments like croquet balls through hoops. The welfare of the patients and the progress of medicine must come first, argued my other colleagues, merely to provoke our retort that good doctoring depends on sound medical education. Thus the controversy swung backwards and forwards until we compromised.

The accident and orthopaedic departments gathered strength at the expense of general surgery. Two more orthopaedic surgeons were added to the staff. General surgery also lost beds to thoracic and plastic surgery, general medicine beds to departments of radiotherapy, physical medicine and psychiatry. But most members of the staff continued to take their share of the ordinary run of patient admissions while carrying on their own particular speciality as a side line.

Large numbers of 'demobbed' doctors, many of whom had been kicking their heels in the services, now wanted to come back to make up for the experience they had missed on account of having qualified during the war. So registrarships, medical and surgical, were duplicated both at the hospital and at the annexe. Numbers of 'demobbed' combatants also now wanted to take up medicine in addition to the normal run of school leavers. So applications for admission to the school soared and, in view of a probable shortage of doctors in a post-war world, I felt compelled to increase the intake of students to the school.

Under these circumstances I remained anxious to retain some of the sector hospitals, where we had built up so much goodwill during the war, for clinical teaching, but on this I was over-ruled by the university element on the college board. That London Hospital students must be taught exclusively by London Hospital teachers seemed to me a narrow view to hold. All students at sector hospitals, where they had lived in at hospital expense and much to their educational advantage, were now withdrawn. Soon they had to be withdrawn from the annexe too because it was impossible to require them to live in Brentwood at their own expense.

'The London' was now crowded with undergraduates and post-graduates and short of beds, both in respect of the demands of patients on our waiting lists and the requirement of teaching. The obvious solution to this problem, it seemed to me, would be to take over Mile End, a municipal hospital less than a mile down the road. (Other hospitals were bent on the same course in respect of municipal hospitals, and for the same reason.) The university recommended it and the LCC, in view of the certain shape of things to come, that is to say, a health service, seemed disposed to play.

Amalgamation with Mile End would be advantageous to 'the London' from the point of view of teaching, and would go a long way towards providing the staff with the beds for which they were clamouring. On the other hand, we were deeply committed to the annexe and it would be difficult to maintain both the annexe and Mile End, in view of the shortage of nurses now prevailing. It was clearly impossible to provide London nurses for both hospitals and to maintain the standards on which matron insisted, so amalgamation would have meant taking on LCC nurses as London Hospital nurses. To this both the matron and the house governor were opposed. It would also have meant taking over LCC doctors who would have to teach 'London' students, at least for a while; a policy to which, as we have seen, there was opposition in academic circles. (The idea that 'the London' should remain completely self-sufficient and its teaching staff for ever undiluted died hard.) It was believed, too, that the damaged wards would soon be repaired and then we would have all the beds we wanted. To blunder into an amalgamation, fraught with so many difficulties and so much opposition, was therefore thought unwise. So the idea of it was allowed to lapse. I felt that a great opportunity had been missed.

The university now started to intrude to an increasing extent into the organization of the medical school. Professorships of surgery and chemical pathology were created. The grant to it, which stood at £15000 in 1939, had been increased to £50000 by 1946 and was now made conditional on the college accepting women, a move still resisted by all the London teaching hospitals. (They had stopped taking women again after the first war.) Direct grants to students were increased and the fees of any ex-servicemen who found a place in a medical school were paid by the state. Generous grants were also now being given by the county councils to school leavers promised places in a medical school. Before long the proportion of students at 'the London' paying their own fees was small, and many whose education was being financed either by local authorities or the state were also in receipt of grants in respect of board and lodgings. In short, medical education was now heavily subsidized both out of the rates and out of the taxpayers' pocket.

Matron had been recentralizing the nursing school. Staff at sector hospitals had been gradually brought back as their services were found redundant and reconstruction in Whitechapel got under way. The units at Warley Woods and Chase Farm, and the maternity unit in Hertfordshire, lingered on longest. Now they came back and the training of nurses was centred entirely on the hospital in Whitechapel and at the annexe in Brentwood, under sister tutors. I gave lectures to them, I remember, in both places.

Miss Alexander, devastatingly efficient but lacking a little in the personal touch – she had been appointed during the war – made many changes. The special 'London' examination, so dear to the heart of Miss Lückes, was dropped and the London Hospital certificate now awarded to every nurse who had spent three years at the hospital and passed the state examination to become a state registered nurse – anathema, it will be recalled, both to Miss Lückes and Miss Nightingale. She also ended the compulsory fourth year. After a nurse's final examination at the end of three years she was now no longer under contract to stay on a fourth in the capacity of staff nurse. Matron had two reasons in mind in making this change. In the first place, many candidates did not want to commit themselves a whole four years ahead and this was adversely affecting recruitment. In the second, it left her free to appoint her staff nurses from among her best student nurses. She also introduced the 'study day'. Hitherto nurses had attended all their classes and lectures in their off-duty time. Now a student nurse spent a whole day every week completely off the wards, and in it attended all her classes and lectures and did her homework. This was followed by a day off. This scheme proved popular. It was copied at other hospitals and served as a valuable stimulus to recruiting at a time when nurses were hard to get, particularly in Whitechapel.

Many of the senior sisters felt unsettled after the war and started asking for a move. To counteract this tendency Miss Alexander introduced a system of three months' leave on full pay after ten years' service. Many of the older sisters, too, were now past the retiring age. They had stayed on to see the hospital through the war. An improved pension scheme made retirement a practical proposition for many. New blood, too, matron could see, was wanted. There had been too much inbreeding for too long and, on her recommendation, the house committee agreed to ten per cent of the nursing staff each year being appointed from other nursing schools.

Miss Alexander had taken over at a difficult time. Nursing was becoming increasingly technical and the social upheaval caused by the war had led to a general questioning of authority at all levels. Her task was certainly no easy one, but it is generally agreed, among those who worked under her, that she was the right person in the right place at the right moment after a series of uninspired appointments. She did much to raise the reputation of the hospital in the outside world. She relaxed the over-rigid standards of behaviour, too long maintained by her predecessors, with dignity and discretion. She gained a reputation for being fair. Her nurses respected her and, where she lacked approachability, the personal touch was supplied by her two assistants, Miss Burgess and Miss Walker. These she had inherited from the old regime.

Great had been the hope of a rapid return to pre-war conditions, but it soon became clear that repairs to damaged buildings would be long delayed by the limitations imposed on the employment of labour, and the use of bricks and mortar by the government. Nothing could now be done without a prior permit from the ministry. Rebuilding the hospital on the estate, as had been envisaged during the phoney war, had long been dismissed as the wildest dream. More serious plans which had been got out later were indefinitely postponed. There was no hope, it seemed, of rebuilding for years to come, but the ministry did promise the governors that they would be allowed to retain the annexe at Brentwood for five years. They also granted permits for the repair and re-equipment of the damaged nurses' homes, and the construction of a new nurses' kitchen and two dining rooms to replace those destroyed by the flying bomb. All the wards were redecorated and the blitzed laundry re-equipped. Flea bites these seemed, out of the oceans that wanted doing. All else had to wait for better times.

It was not only a question of permits either. The hospital had not got the money. 'The London' had finished the last year of the war with a deficit of £22 000, in spite of the fact that income from voluntary subscriptions had in point of fact gone up, due to an all round rise in prices, salaries and wages. This was met by drawing on the legacy account, which had gone up by £63 000. In the following year the deficit proved even greater, in spite of the fact that £53 000 had been received in voluntary subscriptions, largely due to the cost of all the post-war repairs which had been piling up and for which permits had now been obtained. So it was necessary to encroach on the legacy account still further. Now, in the last year of the life of 'the London' as a voluntary hospital, the cost of running it had risen to over six hundred thousand pounds. This was three times as much as it had cost before the war began.

It had in fact now become abundantly clear that the voluntary hospitals would be unable to repair damage done, keep up to date and pay their way without substantial help from the state. So both major political parties had given a national health service a prominent place in their manifestoes in the run up to the general election of 1945. There was nothing novel in the idea. Greece had had one in the fourth century BC, and Sir Thomas More had recommended one in his *Utopia*. Modern opinion, too, had been steadily moving in that direction. Lloyd George's Insurance Act of 1912 had marked the beginning of it; Chamberlain's Local Government Act of 1929 been an extension of it; and now the Emergency Medical Service of 1939 had furthered it. Not only had it been freely discussed during the period of the phoney war, but the Beveridge Commission, appointed by the war-time coalition government, in recommending a comprehensive system of social insurance, had worked on the assumption that a national health service of some kind, covering both domiciliary and hospital treatment, would be introduced.

A number of bodies had been studying the shape it should take. The most important was the Joint Planning Committee of the

British Medical Association, the Royal College of Physicians and the Royal College of Surgeons on which the most influential person was Lord Dawson, now senior physician to 'the London'. He had been President of the Royal College of Physicians since 1938 and, after the debate in the Lords on the Beveridge Report, had been elected President of the British Medical Association for the second time. So when a white paper had been presented to Parliament it had fallen to him, as the acknowledged leader of the profession, to discuss its implications with the coalition government. He died a year later at the age of eighty.

At the general election a swing to the left brought Labour into power and it fell to Aneurin Bevan, an advanced socialist and ardent supporter of the movement for a complete welfare state, now Minister of Health in Attlee's government, to introduce into Parliament a bill to set up a national health service. This, as the result of the strong line taken by the profession in discussions with the minister, proved far less radical than might have been expected and differed little from that which a Conservative government would have introduced, had they been returned to power. A state medical service with state-controlled doctors as in the armed forces, as some had feared, was not contemplated. Mr Bevan respected both the liberty of the patient to choose his doctor and the freedom of the doctor to treat his patients according to his own conscience. He also took the traditions of the hospitals and medical schools, in the light of the way in which they had developed, into serious account.

His Bill passed through both houses of Parliament, the Act taking effect from 5 July 1948. Under it England was divided into twelve regions for the purpose of hospital administration. The governing bodies of the teaching hospitals, consisting hitherto of regular subscribers, were dissolved and replaced by Boards of Governors responsible to the Minister of Health, on which the medical staff, the university, local authorities and other interested outside bodies were represented, under a chairman appointed by the minister. At 'the London', Sir John Mann, who had succeeded Sir William Goschen as chairman, was appointed chairman of the new board, and the house governor, Captain

Brierley, its secretary. All the other hospitals in the north-east region (with the exception of St Bartholomew's as another teaching hospital) were now to be administered by a regional board, its chairman, too, to be appointed by the minister, and on which the governors of the two teaching hospitals in the region were both represented. In this way the work of all the hospitals in the region could be coordinated. The two teaching hospitals occupied a privileged position in the new set-up by virtue of being allowed their own governing bodies directly responsible to the minister.

The entire cost of rebuilding, maintaining, developing and running, including the payment of salaries and wages, was now taken over by the ministry. No longer were patients to be asked to contribute towards their keep. Rich and poor were in future entitled to all their treatment, however expensive, free, and to their board and lodging in hospital, entirely free as well. Hospitals would still make plans for their own development but nothing could be done without the permission of the minister. All major decisions now rested with the ministry who held the purse strings and was now able to control and coordinate the whole hospital system of the country to its best advantage within the limits set by the fraction of the national income allotted to the new health service.

The medical staff were now to be paid for their work more or less in proportion to the time they gave to it. This was the greatest break with tradition to result from the Act. Ever since the foundation of the voluntary hospitals the senior medical staff had given their professional services in a strictly honorary capacity. They had also taught the students allocated to them, as the medical schools developed, without expecting payment of any kind. This, as we have seen, was far from being altruistic on their part. It paid them to do both, and often paid them well, for it was those same students who referred patients to them when themselves in practice later, and it was out of private practice that the honorary staff of the voluntary hospitals contrived their living. As a system it had worked well, fostering loyalty to a hospital and a spirit of cooperation between its old members which had often stood the general public in good stead. Now, on account of economic factors, it was ceasing to work as it had. It had become more and more difficult for a consultant on the staff of a teaching hospital to earn a living. Many now welcomed the prospect of becoming part-time servants of the state.

The teaching hospitals retained their endowment funds. At 'the London' these included income derived from investments and from the estate the purchase of which, now so long ago, had alone rendered expansion of the hospital possible. This could now be spent at the discretion of the new governors on providing amenities for staff and patients. All research funds, too, were to be left untouched and vested in trustees. The college, hitherto run by a committee responsible to the governors of the hospital, was reconstituted under its own board of governors on which the university and the governing body of the hospital were both represented.

While these points were being settled, and these new bodies constituted, the months passed by destitute for most of either anticipation or regret. It would make little difference to their lives. Only members of the house committee and members of the college board, many of whom would now drop out, the honorary staff, now to become part-time servants of the state, and the lawyers and accountants, lived conscious of the coming change. So the days slipped by uncounted and, when the eve of the appointed day arrived, the hours and minutes passed unnoticed. Then the clock struck midnight in the empty board room and John Harrison's hospital, which had endured so much, struggled so hard, even, it can almost be said, fought so well, after the passage of over two hundred years had been taken over by the state.

Next day *The Times* came out with a leading article, painting a rosy picture of the new Health Service. Not a single paper, not even *The Times*, thought fit to publish an obituary of the voluntary hospital system which, after achieving so much, had grown old and finally passed quietly out into history during the previous night.

Epilogue

What was this achievement? The voluntary hospital system bridged the gap in time, in respect of the sick poor in need of hospital treatment, between the dissolution of the religious houses at the Reformation and the institution of the poor-law infirmaries, forced on the state by rapid rise in population in the later part of the nineteenth century. It then continued to provide for most of the acute sick, and to pioneer methods of diagnosis and treatment, until a new political philosophy and the social and economic consequences of two world wars culminated in the Welfare State. This presumes to provide for all the needs of society without recourse to charity.

The voluntary system was the product of private enterprise inspired, not by the pursuit of material gain, but by a crying social need and maintained by charity, that is to say, personal service voluntarily given and financial generosity bred of genuine compassion. Its constituent hospitals were founded mainly by men, lay both in respect of the church and the medical profession. It was in fact these lay governors who not only raised the money, but built them, maintained them, and took all major decisions in respect of them. They also employed the doctors, the leading physicians and surgeons of their day, who served them unpaid from their beginning right up to the coming into force of the National Health Act in 1948.

These physicians and surgeons, as we have seen, served the voluntary hospitals because it was to their advantage; it was not all altruism on their part. Being on the staff of one of the hospitals had become the hallmark of success. Many, however, made great sacrifices on behalf of the particular hospital which they felt it had become their privilege to serve. Many, too, like many of the governors, were also men of enterprise and originality, as the result of which the voluntary hospitals set the pace and maintained the running in respect of the standards of medical practice. These the poor-law infirmaries, later the municipal hospitals, strove to emulate. The medical staff of the voluntary hospitals also founded the medical schools. These, too, were the product of private enterprise inspired by a social need, that of well-trained doctors in society. In fact, just as the voluntary hospitals were started by private enterprise and later taken over by the state, so the medical schools were started by private enterprise and later taken over by the university.

What of the future of the one-time voluntary hospitals? At the time of writing (1978) thirty years of what was future when they were taken over has already run its course. During the first twenty-six of these they carried on under their own boards of governors directly responsible to the Minister of Health, relieved of all necessity to raise money by public appeals and far better off financially than if they had continued under the voluntary system. Without any obligation to any particular area they were now able, within the limits set by their incomes, to cut the *quantity* of their service to the public in order to improve its *quality*, an essential option in any teaching hospital. More affluent as the result of having been taken over by the state, they could continue, with the approval of the ministry, to put *quality* before *quantity* and spend in any particular direction in which the talent of individual members of their staff rendered it worth while.

Four years ago, under the Act of 1974, the Health Service, with which 'the London' had become incorporated in 1948, was reorganized. The boards of governors of the teaching hospitals, set up in 1948, were dissolved and the integration of the work of all the hospitals, both teaching and non-teaching, in the regions handed over to newly constituted regional boards directly responsible to the minister. Our board of governors was now dissolved like all the rest and our chairman became chairman of the north-east regional board. In conjunction with a number of other hospitals we now became responsible to the new regional board for the hospital services in the Tower Hamlets district of

East London. We were also designated the teaching hospital in it, teaching having been officially recognized as a necessary function of most hospitals.

At first sight it may have looked to some as if a severe blow had been struck at private enterprise, which had played such an important part in the history of 'the London', and many are understandably pessimistic as to the future of 'the London' as a continuing entity with an ethos of its own. To me it seems that there need be no fear on this account.

In the first place, we are now in part responsible for the medical services of the district with which we have been long associated, and there is no reason why the health service in action, like an army in the field, should not inspire that sense of service, (in contradistinction to scientific interest in terms of which medicine is taught) just as effectively as the work of the hospitals inspired it in the days of the voluntary system. The motive is the same. It makes no difference where the money comes from.

In the second, our status as a teaching hospital has been officially recognized, and this must strengthen our legal, financial and psychological relationship with the university with which we are now intimately associated and on which we are also financially dependent. The treatment of the sick and the education of doctors are now, it must be remembered, both financed by the state, the two being recognized as mutually interdependent. A large proportion of the clinical staff of the hospital are now full- or part-time servants of the university. Some members of the staff are not only part-time servants both of hospital and college, but are also engaged in part-time private practice. It takes all sorts to make a hospital and medical school.

The school, too, now has its own governing body on which hospital, college, and lay interests are all represented, independent of the university and in no way subservient to it. The amount of money we will get from the state for the development of hospital and college, on the one hand, through the regional board and ministry of health and, on the other, through the university and University Grants Committee, will continued to depend on the wisdom, efficiency and enterprise with which the affairs of both are run in the future, just as much as it depended on that of the house committee and its affiliated college board in the days about which I have been writing.

Thirdly, I believe that charity will and must come back into its own. 'The London' started as a charity, the object of its foundation the care of those 'poor objects'. The major burden of that has now been taken over by the state. But modern medicine has become so expensive that neither the university nor the state can provide everything for everybody. Here it is that charity must step in changing places with the state. Charity must be invoked, not only to look after the poor, but also to endow the health service and the university, pioneering the production or even providing methods of diagnosis and treatment which neither the state nor the university can afford. Only in this way can the teaching hospitals continue those centres of excellence which they became when they gave birth to the medical schools.

'The London' under the voluntary system, which it has been my life's work to serve, which so many of my generation grew to love, and the history of which it has now been my privilege to write, is no more. Nothing like it *could* exist in the modern world. The spirit of the place, I trust, will ever remain unchanged.

Index